HOW TO S
WHEN ENTERING THE
HEALTHCARE SYSTEM

HOW TO STAY SAFE WHEN ENTERING THE HEALTHCARE SYSTEM

A PHYSICIAN WALKS ACROSS THE COUNTRY TO RAISE AWARENESS OF THE NEED TO IMPROVE HEALTHCARE SAFETY

DAVID B. MAYER, MD

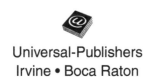

Universal-Publishers
Irvine • Boca Raton

How to Stay Safe When Entering the Healthcare System: A Physician Walks across the Country to Raise Awareness of the Need to Improve Healthcare Safety

Universal Publishers, Inc.
Irvine • Boca Raton
USA • 2022
www.Universal-Publishers.com

ISBN: 978-1-62734-406-7 (pbk.)
ISBN: 978-1-62734-407-4 (ebk.)
ISBN: 978-1-62734-408-1 (audio)

Typeset by Medlar Publishing Solutions Pvt Ltd, India
Cover design by Ivan Popov

Library of Congress Cataloging-in-Publication Data

Names: Mayer, David B., author.
Title: How to stay safe when entering the healthcare system : a physician walks across the country to raise awareness of the need to improve healthcare safety / David B. Mayer, MD.
Description: Irvine : Universal Publishers, 2022. | Includes bibliographical references.
Identifiers: LCCN 2022024984 (print) | LCCN 2022024985 (ebook) | ISBN 9781627344067 (paperback) | ISBN 9781627344074 (ebook)
Subjects: LCSH: Medical errors--United States--Prevention--Popular works. | Medical care--United States--Quality control--Popular works. | Health facilities--United States--Safety measures--Popular works. | Health care reform--United States--Popular works.
Classification: LCC R729.8 .M39 2022 (print) | LCC R729.8 (ebook) | DDC 362.1028/9--dc23/eng/20220708
LC record available at https://lccn.loc.gov/2022024984
LC ebook record available at https://lccn.loc.gov/2022024985

Table of Contents

Acknowledgments

To all the patients, family members, healthcare workers, and friends who walked with me in memory of loved ones lost due to preventable medical harm. You kept my spirits high and provided energy on days I was dragging: Lisa Riegle, Barbara Black, Vonda Vaden-Bates, Carole Hemmelgarn, Lee Perreira, Dr. Art Kanowitz, Shelley Dierking, Dr. Wendy Madigosky, Tracy Pierce, Josh Pierce, Ellie Pierce, Lainey Pierce, Deahna Visscher, Marty Hatlie, Tracy Granzyk, Steve Burrows, Margo Burrows, Soojin Jun, Greg Vass, Dr. Tim McDonald, Brad Schwartz, Chrissie Blackburn, Katie Carlin, Crystal Morales, Dr. Delbert Morales, Jack Gentry, Teresa Gentry, Dr. Raj Ratwani, Leah Binder, Armando Nahum, Angela Nahum, Debbie Zelinski, Brian Zelinski, Tony Galbo, Liz Galbo, Michelle Bennett, Joe Kiani, Ariana Longley, Dr. Bill Wilson, and Bernadette Wilson.

To my wife Cathy who walked with me cross-country while also serving as our sag wagon leader. Without her love and support, I would have never finished.

To my mother Charlotte who died too early, never experiencing the love and joy that comes with being a grandparent.

To my father Ben and my sister Debbie whose lives were shortened by preventable harm.

To my children and grandchildren—I am so blessed and proud of all of you.

To Tracy Granzyk and Terry Ratner who helped shape this book's narrative through their outstanding writing skills and story-telling abilities.

To Steve Evans, CMO, Ken Samet, CEO, and Larry Smith, VP of Risk Management at MedStar Health. Thank you for trusting my leadership, supporting our quality and safety efforts through the years, and fully embracing open and honest communication after preventable medical harm across our health system. I have been fortunate to work for an amazing healthcare system.

To Janice Wagner, Arnold Meisner, and Inez Meisner who helped support me when I was still trying to find my way.

To Dr. Tim McDonald for his 30-plus years of friendship, mentorship, leadership, and partnership in our numerous patient safety efforts.

To Rosemary Gibson who taught me the value of story-telling while sharing a vision of empathic and transparent healthcare for all.

My walk across America:

1. Walked 2,460 miles over 355 consecutive days during the pandemic.
2. Interviewed by over seventy-five television, radio, newspaper, and podcast outlets including *The Washington Post*, *Chicago Tribune*, NPR, PBS and ESPN sports radio programs, raising awareness about the preventable harm crisis in healthcare.
3. Walked to 20 Major League Ballparks, fourteen spring training ballparks, and three minor league ballparks.
4. Drove 13,368 miles while visiting twenty-six different states.
5. Raised over $40,000 for the Patient Safety Movement Foundation.
6. Used twelve pairs of Brooks running shoes over the course of the year.
7. Suffered two broken toes, recurrent back spasms, and associated hip and knee pains.

"To err is human, to cover-up is unforgivable, to fail to learn
is inexcusable."

Sir Liam Donaldson, Former Chief Medical Officer for England

I learned how to lie to patients during my third year of residency.

It was a simple surgery in 1985, a routine hernia repair on the right side
of the patient's abdomen. I remember when I first greeted James Wilson in
the preop holding area that morning and commented on his classic thick
mop-like-style 'stache, which resembled a black caterpillar covering his upper
lip, reminiscent of Tom Selleck from *Magnum PI*. Although fifty-six years of
age, his lean muscular physique reflected many years of working in construction, the heavy lifting adding to his weakened abdominal wall. The patient
appeared relaxed and knowledgeable about his procedure—one that our surgical teams performed hundreds of times during a year. The thought this case
would be any different never crossed my mind.

Mr. Wilson and I chatted about his anesthetic plan and the routine one-
hour stay in the recovery room after surgery. After verifying his lab work and
pre-operative tests were within normal range, he signed the anesthesia consent
for treatment. "We'll take good care of you," I told him before administering
a rapid-acting sedative through his intravenous line. When his eyes began to
close I went to my usual place at the head of the bed, unlocked the brakes, and
began pushing the steel-framed bed down the hallway toward the operating
rooms of our university hospital. Once through the wooden double doors,
I made my way past two cardiac and neurosurgical rooms where cases were
already being prepped. By the time we arrived at the general surgery room we
were assigned to, Mr. Wilson had fallen into a light sleep.

Once inside, I roused him gently and helped him off the gurney and
then on to the surgical bed. I secured him to the table by stretching a leather
belt across his waist—one of the safety protocols we had in place at the time.

Over the years, a few mildly sedated patients had been injured after rolling over and falling off the operating room table while OR staff were preoccupied preparing for the case. The safety strap was on the mental checklist I ran through before each case began. The next steps involved connecting his blood pressure cuff, heart monitor, and pulse oximeter. It was standard procedure to double-check the patient's vital signs one last time before administering sodium pentothal, a rapid-acting induction agent we used back in the mid-eighties to induce unconsciousness, and succinylcholine, a paralytic agent that allowed me to take control of his airway.

I would continue to record his heart rate, blood pressure, oxygen saturation, and temperature every five minutes, critical vital signs required by the American Society of Anesthesiologists guidelines, until the procedure ended. Double-checking every detail had been ingrained early in my career when I found one of my monitors unplugged by the cleaning staff who sterilized OR rooms between cases. Anesthesiologists joke that our job consists of hours of boredom and moments of terror, something none of us wanted to experience. Satisfied his monitors were working correctly, I injected the anesthetic medications that would put Mr. Wilson to sleep. When he reached a deep state of unconsciousness and I had secured control of his breathing, I let the surgical team know we were ready to begin.

Once we had the case under control, my supervising anesthesiologist left the operating room. I settled in on the metal stool at the head of the table behind the paper drape protecting the sterile surgical field from the anesthesia work area. For the next forty-five minutes, my job entailed checking monitors, charting vital signs, and recording any drugs given during the procedure.

The surgical team sprang into action prepping and draping the patient. The faster we completed each case, the more cases we could perform in a day. At times it felt like we were more concerned about tracking profits than we were patient outcomes. With Mr. Wilson stable, I documented the required comments about proper placement of his breathing tube, which I verified by placing my stethoscope on each side of his chest, listening for the subtle swoosh of air filling each lung through mechanical ventilation. I noted that his eyes were lubed and taped shut to avoid corneal abrasions, since patients cannot blink while paralyzed, and that we did not chip any of his teeth when we intubated him—all obligatory details to protect the hospital in the event of a lawsuit.

While I was documenting details, I heard the senior surgical resident announce, "Incision made," a routine phrase I had heard hundreds of times indicating the official surgical start time for circulating nurses and anesthesiologists to record in their medical records. Mr. Wilson's vital signs remained normal after the incision and I was content that his depth of anesthesia was correct. I returned to my record keeping, confident all was good.

Two minutes into the surgery, the surgical attending arrived and glanced at Mr. Wilson's operative site. "I thought this was a right-sided inguinal hernia repair?"

The resident looked down at her incision, and traced the red line left by her scalpel on Mr. Wilson's left side. Color drained from her face as she dropped to one knee at the side of the operating table. She realized her mistake.

I stood up and stared at the wrong-sided surgical incision, unsure of how I should respond. My reflex was to check the patient's vital signs, which remained normal, unlike my own heart rate and blood pressure, which I'm certain had soared waiting for the wrath of the attending surgeon. Except for the steady beeping of the patient's heart rate on the pulse oximeter, I still remember the eerie silence in the room. No one said a word while we helped the stunned surgical resident to a chair in the corner of the room.

I made my way back to the head of the operating table, wanting to disappear behind the drape to pretend that I had nothing to do with the error. The shame and blame culture of our medical profession guaranteed it would only be a matter of time before our team suffered the consequences of our error. Despite what I believed to be a keen attention to detail and safety, I failed to keep my patient safe.

I wondered how this medical error might damage my professional career. Would I be disciplined by the hospital, suspended by the department, or face criminal charges? I then focused my thoughts and concern back on what had occurred minutes ago in the operating room with my patient.

Every resident physician is conditioned early in training that someone is at fault when things go wrong. Before being indoctrinated into the culture, we believed the ABCs of medicine referred to "Airway, Breathing, Circulation." Once in the line of fire, we found out it really meant: "Assess Blame Correctly." This was the cutthroat culture that prevented honesty and truthfulness in medicine, and it was something none of us wanted to be a target of at any point in our career. I now found myself in that position. The fear in my heart was etched upon my face, only partially hidden by my sterile mask. Silence filled the room during the rest of the procedure.

Mr. Wilson's surgery continued uneventfully from there; the team was in shock but taking even more care with each finishing step. The attending surgeon and junior surgical resident closed the left-side incision and proceeded to repair his right-sided hernia. Surgical dressings were placed on both incisions, calling attention to our error. There would be no hiding our mistake, which is often the first strategy hospitals use when medical errors are made. When the attending made his last stitch, he left the operating room without saying a word.

It was now my responsibility to take our patient to the recovery room and give an update on his status to the nurse who would take over his care. Wheeling him down the hallway, I wondered who had already found out about what we had done. News travels fast in hospitals, especially bad news and gossip. The thought that I might be forever labeled by this error made me nauseous. I handed Mr. Wilson off to the recovery room team and went back to the operating room to clean up, still unable to look at anyone. Now all I could think about was having to discharge him. His trusting, tentative face just hours earlier came to mind, and my reassurance that we would take good care of him felt like empty words. I knew he would be expressing anger, not the usual gratitude a patient feels after coming out of anesthesia.

The hour waiting to discharge Mr. Wilson remains one of the longest hours of my life. When the nurse paged me, I took several deep breaths before heading toward the recovery room. To my amazement, he greeted me with a smile when I entered the room.

"Today is my lucky day!"

Dumbfounded, I said nothing.

"My surgeon told me he discovered a second hernia on my left side and was able to fix both. I don't need to miss a second day of work."

I was speechless. Thoughts raced through my mind. Should I be honest with him? Should I tell him what had really happened? The consequences for contradicting an attending, for being honest and open about what had occurred, could be career ending for a resident. Everything inside me—what I knew of right and wrong, how I had been raised, who I was as a person, a doctor—was being tested. My inner voice wanted to shout the truth. But instead, like those before me and after, I followed the leader who told the first lie and buried the truth.

"Yes, today is your lucky day," I replied. And I signed him out of the recovery room.

Thirty-five years later, this error and the lies that followed still haunt me. Like many of my colleagues, I have been fighting for a safer healthcare system for three decades, one that does not lose 250,000 patients each year to preventable medical harm. One that does not have healthcare workforce injuries, depression, suicide, and burnout rates higher than almost every other industry. After spending a significant portion of my professional career trying to improve patient safety, not much had changed. Yes, we were better able to quantify our bad outcomes, but the serious safety-event numbers have shown little improvement. Hundreds of lectures and keynote presentations around the world, sharing tools and techniques that could reduce patient risk in hospitals, sitting on advisory boards and patient safety committees working with others to make healthcare safer—this had been my life's work and we were still far from protecting patients and healthcare professionals from the same harm, occurring over and over again.

So, in late February of 2020, I decided to approach this intractable problem from a different angle. I would do something outrageous to draw public attention to the current healthcare safety crisis. At sixty-seven years of age, while being treated for thyroid and prostate cancer, I outlined a plan to walk across America using my love for baseball and the Major League Baseball stadiums as anchors that I hoped would draw media attention to my mission.

With voice recorder in hand, I set out to raise awareness of the need to improve healthcare safety by sharing stories of family members who had lost loved ones to preventable medical harm, many who walked with me as I passed through their hometowns. Little did I know we would experience the worst pandemic in over a century shortly after I began my walk on February 28th in San Diego. When the world exploded around me, I documented the political divide and social unrest I witnessed. The prejudice I experienced along the way forced me to revisit my Jewish upbringing and the role it played not only in shaping my mission, but also in helping me to achieve my goal during a year like none other in our country's history.

"History can teach us that human actions have consequences, and
that certain choices, once made, cannot be undone."

Gerda Lerner

My mother, Charlotte, always wanted me to become a doctor. I wanted to
be a professional baseball player. It was her dream to see me in a white coat
helping others in need. It was my dream to wear Cubs pinstripes.

Her desire for a doctor in the family seemed ironic since she never trusted
physicians. She had been diagnosed with diabetes during her early twenties
and within a few years diagnosed with a connective tissue disease. The gene
for autoimmune disorders ran deep throughout her side of our family, and
two of her brothers also lived with diabetes from an early age. Mom and my
two closest uncles, Irv and Lou, were constantly taking shots at physicians
during family gatherings or holidays, her older brother Lou leading a constant
refrain of "... they're all quacks ... always sending me for more tests that never
help me feel better." Uncle Lou's tirades became much harsher as he aged, his
physical discomfort fueling his resigned disgust. "Ah, fuck 'em. Fuck 'em all!"
he'd say, swatting at the air. Mom would also chime in but was never one to
complain directly to her doctors. She would wait until after they had exited
her hospital room or she had left their office to resume her rants.

My dad, Ben, was an optimist, and more introspective than my mother.
He loved to swim and even quit smoking at the age of thirty-five after hearing
about the potential health issues connected to the addicting plant that put
North Carolina on the agricultural map. On Friday nights he mixed himself
a Beefeater gin martini straight up with three olives, joking that his doctor
prescribed it to help him relax and unwind after a long work week. He was
bone thin yet carried the weight of my mother's physical ailments. Dad served
as a buffer between her constant pain and his children's discomfort watching
their mother suffer each day. He was the one who tried to stay positive, gently

challenging Mom's wariness of her doctors. "Let them try, Char," he'd say. "Listen to what they say. Give them a chance to do their job."

Her complex autoimmune diseases caused dizzy spells and neurological symptoms that had her doctors shaking their heads and throwing their arms up in the air. Because of her diabetes, any foot injury was a major concern for infection and all of her complaints of chest pain required an immediate trip to the emergency room. Over time, the increasing fatigue in Dad's eyes exposed the burden he carried, but he never complained.

I grew up in a Jewish community—Skokie, Illinois—surrounded by Jewish families. My friends and I joked that all parents wanted their children to become either doctors, lawyers, or accountants. Not only were these well-respected professions that required dedication to higher learning, but they also provided a good living for families, all qualities our community valued.

As a child, I lived and breathed sports. If I wasn't on the baseball diamond, I'd be shooting hoops at the neighborhood park after school or watching ballgames that aired on the weekend or played during the week. I couldn't get enough baseball—an addiction that stayed with me for life. School was somewhere I had to be, but the baseball diamond was somewhere I dreamed of being. If I wasn't at a local park with my glove waiting for a pickup game to begin, I was relaxing in our basement watching a Cubs game on the old black-and-white, twelve-inch RCA Victor TV.

One afternoon after an emotional, but expected, Cubby loss, I started up the basement steps to finish my homework but stopped midway when I heard my mother and her friends chatting over the familiar clatter of mahjong tiles. Each mother was taking a turn bragging about her son or daughter.

"Steven is going to be a doctor. I've had dreams of seeing him in a long white coat so I know it will happen," said one mother who lived down the street.

A friend from our synagogue spoke up. "Michelle will study law. She is a born debater."

My mother didn't hesitate to add to the chorus of proud parents. "David will be a great doctor. He's so kind and caring, and his teachers are always complimenting his science and math skills."

Her excitement and pride echoed down the stairs and caught me by surprise. My life up to now revolved around playing and watching sports. I dreamt about playing center field for the Cubs, chasing down fly balls, and hitting dingers, not trying to cure the incurable. The one thing I knew for sure is that I wanted my mother to be proud of me.

My parents were first-generation Americans—raised to make a better life for their children. All four of my grandparents were Russian Jews who came to the United States in 1920 from Kyiv shortly after World War I ended. By then, the open door for immigrants was becoming more restrictive, especially for those who were ill, uneducated, or who were not successful professionals.

A visit with my grandparents Samuel and Rose gave me, at the age of eight, a glimpse into their lives back in Kyiv where they were born and raised. My father's parents were in their late seventies by then, and lived on the second floor of a three-story, brick walk-up apartment building in Rogers Park, a predominantly Jewish neighborhood on the north side of Chicago. Their one-bedroom apartment smelled of moth balls, the odor so pungent I often held my breath as I followed my parents through the front door. Manischewitz candles in clear glass jars burned atop furniture and cabinets in the living room and kitchen, an old Jewish tradition. The white candles were lit as a memorial, or *Yahrzeit*, on the anniversary of a family member's death. My grandparents also used them as everyday candles, adding new ones for *Yahrzeit* reasons and making their living space feel like a dimly lit shrine honoring the dead.

I was convinced my grandfather never left the apartment. He always donned the same gray cuffed trousers held up by suspenders over a white button-down shirt that covered a sleeveless undershirt, and remained planted in his high-backed, cushioned armchair in the living room reading the daily news and obituaries through wire-rimmed glasses. An old Western movie played in the background on their small black-and-white television. The only time I ever saw him leave his chair was at lunchtime to join my grandmother in the kitchen where she had prepared a traditional Russian lunch of beet borscht with sour cream, warmed up brisket or fish from the previous night's supper or chicken soup.

At five feet tall and eighty-five pounds at most, my grandmother appeared frail. For our weekly visit she dressed in her Sunday best: a faded, floral scooped-neck dress that fell to her ankles, her curly grey hair pulled up off her neck with a rubber band. She wore identical wire-rimmed glasses as my grandfather and shuffled around the apartment in old slippers catering to his every need, along with ours. Watching her struggle moving from room to room, it was hard to believe she pushed a metal cart three blocks to the grocery store and back every few days no matter the season. Rogers Park was a few blocks from the Chicago lakefront where biting northern winds picked up speed over the water hitting land with enough force to push someone twice her size off course.

They seemed lonely confined to their candle-lit apartment. All their friends had passed away, and my parents told me how special our visits were to them despite the fact they often fell asleep watching TV while we were there. It felt like a waste of a day off from school, especially when the adults spoke Yiddish, which I didn't understand. It sounded like a jumble of consonants that I couldn't begin to comprehend—a guttural alien-sounding language. I also sensed they were talking about things they didn't want me to understand. What little I could make out of their conversations revolved around friends who had died and how hard it was to grow old. I struggled in their presence. My innate shyness combined with the seventy-year age gap and the language barrier made conversation between us forced. Mom would do her best to pull a few words out of me, trying to facilitate communication across decades of cultural differences. "Tell Grandma and Grampa about your week at school," she'd say. "It was fine," was the best I could do—the conversation ending before it began.

On a Sunday afternoon while visiting, both bored and curious, I wandered into my grandparents' bedroom. Once my eyes adjusted to the darkness, I was drawn to a commanding oval-shaped picture of my grandfather wearing a formal military uniform decorated with medals that hung above a large mahogany dresser. He looked stately, youthful, and strong, and I wondered why no one had told me my grandfather had been a military leader. Neither of my grandparents talked about their lives before coming to America, and even at eight years old, I could feel a ripple of discomfort whenever they were asked about it. I went back to the living room determined to ask questions. I wondered about that man in the photo. What was the story behind the uniform?

When I returned to the living room, Grandpa was sitting in his recliner, sleeping with his mouth half open. When he woke, Yiddish spilled out and the room became filled with familiar yet foreign words. I was left wondering about the backstory—too scared to initiate the conversation. And besides, I didn't know how to speak Yiddish.

My grandfather died one month after that visit. Three weeks after his death, my grandmother pointed to a cardboard box in the corner of the living room and said: "I'm going to die very soon. I don't want to live without Shmuel," Shmuel being the Yiddish name for Samuel. "All our keepsakes, anything we have of value, is in that box. Do what you want with it."

4

Her statement upset my parents, who insisted she was talking nonsense and that she was fine. Like she predicted, my grandmother died that night in her sleep, taking the stories of their lives in Russia with her. While I'll never know if it was my grandfather's military position, the fact that they were Jewish, or a specific injustice they suffered because of the antisemitic pogroms that prompted them to leave their homeland, I do know that they had learned, like others, to remain silent about the past.

A Love of Baseball

2

"It's a great day for a ball game; let's play two!"

Ernie Banks, Chicago Cubs Hall of Fame Shortstop

Our family had settled in Skokie, Illinois, just north of Chicago's city limits in 1956. My parents rented near Mom's brothers a two-story, red-brick town-home with two bedrooms and a small patch of grass that passed for a front yard. Compared to our previous one-bedroom apartment in West Rogers Park, the townhome felt like a castle.

The community was only a few years old, but it was quickly becoming a typical middle-class, Midwestern suburb with a large Jewish population. At the time, Skokie was believed to have the largest number of Holocaust survivors in the world outside of Israel. My parents kept the details of the Holocaust horrors suffered by friends of our family secrets from my sister Debbie and me. While their intention was to protect us, the continued chain of secrets left us both insulated from the painful truths my friends and their families suffered because of the Holocaust.

In 1959, when I was six, my parents walked me across the alley mid-afternoon to spend the night with my Aunt Jean and Uncle Lou. I had never stayed overnight with them before but was excited to stay up late watching TV with my two older cousins. With a kiss good night, they promised to pick me up the following morning. When they showed up the next day, my mother was holding a baby girl in her arms. My new little sister, Debbie, was bundled in a pink cotton blanket and my mom encouraged me to say hello while the adults fawned over the newest addition to our family. My parents talked about how lucky I was to have a sister and how important it was to be a good big brother and to look out for her.

I peered over my mom's arms and took in Debbie's chubby little face, immediately excited to have a sibling. But even at six years old, I was caught off guard. I was too young to fully comprehend that they had kept how she was conceived a secret from me, but old enough to understand there had not been any discussion about my mother being pregnant, or that I would be waking up taking on the role of big brother. There were questions I wanted to ask but didn't.

Later that summer, my father took me to my first Chicago Cubs baseball game at Wrigley Field, or "The Friendly Confines," as Ernie Banks called it. It was one of those picture-perfect Chicago afternoons—mild temperatures in the low eighties, blue skies with a few white clouds, and a light breeze blowing out of the south toward left field. I brought my new orange-colored Wilson baseball glove, loving the smell of fresh leather when I lifted the mitt up to my face. The mitt was two sizes too big for my six-year-old hand but that didn't bother me. Along with the blue Cubs cap my dad had bought for me earlier that week to celebrate the occasion, I was out of bed at 7:00am that Saturday morning, dressed and ready to go. We arrived at the ballpark as the gates opened to the public and I quickly ran up the concrete stairs leading to the left field bleachers. Back then, bleacher seats were first-come, first-served, and I wanted to make sure we had good seats in time for batting practice.

Finding seats about ten rows up from the left field wall, I stood the entire batting practice session, never taking my eye off the batter in the batting cage, ready for that special moment when a fly ball would clear the ivy-covered left field wall and land in my mitt. Many baseballs made it into the bleachers during batting practice but not one landed in my mitt. The Cubs lost the ballgame that day, as was so often the case in those years. Despite not catching a baseball and the Cubs losing, the day was perfect. I was officially hooked on baseball and the Chicago Cubs, becoming an annual summer passenger on the Skokie Swift and Chicago Transit Authority elevated trains. After exiting the train at the Addison Street stop, my friends and I walked the one block to Wrigley Field, finding our spot in the left field bleachers.

It wasn't until I was fifteen that I saw my first Holocaust tattoo while visiting a friend. He introduced me to his parents, and when his dad reached out to shake my hand, I saw the telltale numbers tattooed on his forearm. I was still somewhat naïve to the assault and battery it implied, not having anyone in my immediate family who shared the same scarring. I asked my friend about it, to see if maybe someone my age might be more willing to tell me the truth. He too was practiced in the silent nature of our culture, and said, "My parents never talk about it." I let it go, understanding his discomfort all too well. We settled in to watch the Cubs on television, welcoming the silent camaraderie afforded by professional sports. Suddenly and without prompting, my friend changed his mind and confided that his father had spent time in one of Adolf Hitler's concentration camps. The tattoo on his forearm was a life-long branding, a constant reminder of the terrible acts he had survived and the deaths he had witnessed.

Because my parents didn't go to college, they made Debbie's and my high school and college education a top priority. I had never been a hard-working student during high school; things like math and science were easy A's with little study needed on my part. I liked the immediate gratification of finding the correct answer. Subjects like history and language arts, however, were more challenging in their ambiguity. I was uninterested in subjects that did not have concrete solutions. Grammar rules that were hard to grasp and being forced to read books I didn't find interesting made those classes more difficult. Instead of studying harder to improve my grades in those classes, I preferred to grab my baseball mitt or a basketball and head to Oakton Community Center Park for a pick-up game. I wasn't a straight-A student, but I did enough work to remain academically competitive while also having plenty of time to play and watch the sports I loved.

Team sports like baseball, basketball, and football were, and remain, my passion. The synergies that come from great teamwork, the sum of the parts being greater than any individual player, took the game to a higher level for me. I was ultra-competitive and hated to lose, often stretching the rules to my advantage in order to win. While I wasn't tall or a particularly gifted athlete, I worked hard and hustled, using every inch of my five foot, eleven inch frame to gain an edge over my opponent. In basketball, I played aggressive defense, perfecting the fundamentals of stance and positioning, keeping on the balls of my feet, eyes on the belt, hands up, ready for anything. When overmatched against taller opponents under the boards, I wasn't above stepping on their Converse high tops at just the right time, giving me a chance for the rebound while they tried to get out from under me.

Basketball coaches appreciated my tenacity despite my paltry scoring average. During one high school varsity game, we were getting slaughtered by one of the best teams in the state. I was a junior and played limited minutes, mostly when the game was out of reach. We were midway through the second quarter when our coach looked down the bench and yelled my name. Startled, I jumped up and ran toward him, tripping over my warm-up suit while trying to take it off.

"I don't care if you foul out," he said. "We need someone to play hard nose defense and make them earn their points."

Two minutes and forty-three seconds later, I was whistled for my fifth foul, which spurred a skirmish on court before I took my place back at the end of the bench. At halftime, our coach approached me in the locker room and thanked me for my effort with a chuckle. At the end of practice the following day, our assistant coach pulled us together.

"We may have had our asses handed to us on the court yesterday," he said, "but Mayer set a record for fouling out quicker than anyone in a Suburban League high school basketball game." The team erupted in laughter, a bunch of the guys slapping me on the back.

"A little heart goes a long way," he added before walking back to his office. I knew only one way to play sports, and that was to compete to the best of my ability every moment I had a chance to prove myself. The competitive drive and spirit were innate and served me well. It kept me perpetually moving forward, no matter the circumstances around me.

Compared to my father's parents, the relationship I had with my maternal grandmother was warmer. My mom's father died when I was two years old, but her mother, whom we called Bubby Cupcake, lived into my high school years. She was approachable, had a sense of humor, and was so nicknamed because she would steal bites of holiday cupcakes before they were served for dessert. She was also the only living relative I had who spoke Russian.

In my freshman year of high school I decided to take Russian to fulfill my four-year foreign language requirement. I thought it would help me better understand what my grandparents had lived through before coming to America, since no one wanted to talk about it. About a month after starting my Russian class, we were visiting my Uncle Irv's home where Bubby Cupcake lived. She was sitting in the living room by herself watching TV while the rest of the adults were in the kitchen having coffee and cake. I had tired of watching the younger girls play with their dolls in the basement and sat down next to her. She smiled and asked how school was going.

"I love my Russian class," I said, excited to tell her about something we had in common. "It's so different from my general classes. I feel like I'm learning more about where our family came from too."

"*Dobriy den!*" Good afternoon, she said, her smile brightening.

"*Dobriy den,*" I replied.

She continued in Russian, the words flowing from her tongue with ease just like my teacher at school. I laughed, realizing four weeks of Russian tempered my ability but not my enthusiasm to talk with her. The few words I could recall sounded more American with a heavy Chicago accent, but Bubby Cupcake didn't try to correct or criticize my early attempts. I continued to throw out words still fresh in my mind, not wanting the exchange to end.

"*Biblioteka* means library," I said proudly. "*Shkola* is school." I searched for words. "*Kak dela?*" How are you? I asked. Once again, her rapid-fire answer exceeded my still-forming vocabulary, but I could see the joy on her face while being able to share her native language with me.

"I hope we can continue to speak Russian together as you learn more," she said. I nodded and felt a deeper bond forming between us.

"Bubby, I'm learning so much about what Russia is like today, but what was it like when you and Grandpa lived there?"

Her smile faded and her gaze left me, finding the wall on the other side of the room. It was as if she'd seen a ghost and couldn't bear to allow it into the room by talking about it. I had seen the same response from many others in our community when the past was raised in conversation. After a heavy pause she said, "It was not good. It was why we left."

I didn't want to make her uncomfortable, so I never asked her again. Her death during my senior year in high school was a great loss in a year that would prove to be filled with major life transitions. And though my questions about the past may have stopped, my need to understand only intensified. I began reading books about Stalin, Lenin, Trotsky, Tolstoy, and the Bolshevik Revolution in high school, intent on educating myself about what our family's history may have looked like.

One thing our family could not avoid as easily as the past was my mother's chronic illness and pain. I was seventeen when she was hospitalized with chronic lymphocytic leukemia (CLL) in 1970 and I remember visiting her with my father the second night she was in the hospital. I can still picture how fragile and scared Mom looked lying in her hospital bed wearing the flimsy gray-and-white hospital gown. It had only been two days, but she appeared to have aged five years since I last saw her leaving the house with my father on their way to the hospital. My dad wasn't one to reveal his emotions, and though the doctors assured us that CLL was the "good type" of leukemia, the fear on my father's face and the questions he would ask made me think that whatever was going on with Mom must be serious.

Her primary care physician, oncologist, rheumatologist, and nurses told my dad people with CLL can live for twenty years or more. My mother didn't believe any of the doctors. Even encouraging news about lab results and X-ray findings were suspect. As soon as they left her room, she told all of us with conviction that she had only a few months to live. I didn't know whom or what to believe. The doctors seemed like they were being truthful and had no reason to lie or sugar-coat their findings. But it was leukemia, and it was my mother, and it all sounded frightening.

At the foot of her bed hung a gray metal clipboard, the file cabinet of old school medicine. Inside was her handwritten medical chart, which included current and past medical history. The medical chart was available for anyone visiting to pick up and read. Hanging the medical record at the foot of the bed made it easy for physicians to find charts during rounds, a convenient strategy making patient privacy a secondary concern.

With Mom telling us she was going to die despite her doctors' positive prognosis, I wanted to understand what was wrong with her. By now, I had grown wary of my family's secretive nature and had developed a coping method of my own amid all the ambiguity. I taught myself to seek as much information as I could find on topics no one in my family wanted to discuss.

That evening I found myself alone in her hospital room while she slept. My father had left to call her brother, and I quietly picked up her thick chart. I began flipping through the pages, reading what the doctors and nurses had written about her illness and long-term survival. I found myself mesmerized by the medical jargon, a precise language all of its own, which like Russian or Yiddish needed to be studied, memorized, and acted upon. When I reached the section that contained her past medical and surgical history, I stopped short. In the text was noted: "Hysterectomy, November 1952." I re-read the date to make sure I wasn't mistaken. I had been born in March of 1953, four months after this surgery. This could only mean that I had been adopted, like my sister.

I had picked up her medical record, looking for information about the present, not the past. This fact, laid out in cold, black ink confirmed doubts I had carried about my birthright that had begun when I was ten years old. I didn't look like either of my parents, and when I told my friends' parents that I was Jewish, many were quick to tell me, "You don't look Jewish." Combined with my sister's sudden arrival and my mother never having appeared pregnant, and cryptic comments tossed out at family parties, there was evidence that both Debbie and I had been adopted.

I was still processing this information when my father walked back into the room. I wasn't sure it was the right time to confront him with my mother lying in a hospital bed believing she was dying. Dad had so much on his plate, managing Mom's illnesses, keeping her brothers and sisters up to date, talking with doctors, and working long hours. Discussion about my adoption, like so many other secrets in my life, would have to wait for now.

Little did I know then that the secrecy I had grown up with would lead me to become a staunch national advocate for a healthcare system that is not secretive, but one that is fully transparent and embraces open and honest communication.

What I also didn't realize during my teenage years was my mother's illnesses and hospitalizations were preparing me for a career in medicine, what she had always hoped for. It was as if my high school major was health care. Through her struggles, I gained an appreciation of the growing number of medical specialties that existed, and the medical tests and procedures used to arrive at a medical diagnosis, and I began to understand the role and the hierarchy of doctors, nurses, pharmacists, and medical residents.

I also learned that physicians did not have all the answers.

Secrets

3

"Our death is not an end if we can live on in our children and the younger generation. For they are us; our bodies are only wilted leaves on the tree of life."

Albert Einstein

When I left for college, my parents relocated to Fort Lauderdale, Florida, hoping that the milder weather would be easier on Mom. In the spring of 1978, after applying to a handful of medical schools, I received a letter of acceptance from the Abraham Lincoln School of Medicine at the University of Illinois. The school was my first choice because it was a top-rated clinical medical school and the in-state tuition costs were markedly less than those of a private medical school. My mother's dream for her son to study medicine was now a reality. What she didn't know then was the enormous impact her ongoing health issues would have on my career in improving patient care and accountability at every level of our healthcare system. I had witnessed years of good care, as well as inadequate care and misguided treatments. Those experiences helped change the direction of my medical practice. Becoming a doctor was my mother's dream. Now it had become my dream as well.

One early summer day near the end of my third year of medical school, my dad returned from work to find my mother sitting in her chair, wearing the same nightgown and slippers she had on when he had left for work nine hours earlier. She was confused and couldn't remember who or where she was. He called me that evening from the emergency department with news that CT and MRI scans revealed mom had glioblastoma, a malignant and highly aggressive brain tumor. I could hear the devastation and fear in his voice as he shared the day's events, initially thinking she had a small stroke, only to be told she had another cancer.

My first reaction was shock. How much more suffering could she take?

He let me know she was being admitted to the hospital and he would be staying with her overnight before hanging up the phone when we could no longer bear the silence between us. We were each in our own worlds trying to cope with the inevitable.

After hanging up the phone, shock turned to denial. In my second year of medical school, I learned that Kubler-Ross defined the five stages of grief patients go through when learning they have cancer—denial, anger, bargaining, depression, and acceptance. While it was my mother's cancer, I now found myself in the first stage—denial. "Maybe it was a mistake, maybe the radiologist read the scan wrong and it was a benign tumor." I had observed during my clinical rotations that doctors aren't always right. There are often misconstrued test results. My denial soon became short-lived, having learned in my young medical career that it's difficult to misinterpret the characteristic signs of a glioblastoma tumor on a CT scan.

Thoughts and emotions continued racing through my mind, my training as a young but still unlicensed caregiver, telling me I had to study everything I could about glioblastoma. My mother needed me to find a possible cure or at least ensure she received the best care possible while being ushered through an army of doctors and different treatment plans. My father would also lean heavily on me as he had done in the past, looking for answers to the many difficult decisions that lay ahead. I now was petrified, wondering how I would manage it all.

The name and face of Butch Nelson suddenly entered my mind. His real name was William Nelson but he wanted everyone to call him "Butch," not Mr. Nelson, joking that Mr. Nelson was his father.

I was two days into my third year of medical school, dressed appropriately in a freshly pressed white lab coat visiting patients on the medical-surgical floor when I first met Butch. Butch was a smoker in his late fifties diagnosed with laryngeal cancer. He had a rounded, bulging chest resembling a barrel and his wheezes were audible without using a stethoscope. His pale skin had deep lines engraved around his mouth with dark hair slicked back, looking wet and glistening when the sun came through his window. His treatment plan included radiation to shrink the growth in his throat so that his oncologic surgeon could resect the tumor. Being early in my clinical career, my clinical interactions with patients were limited. I believed senior residents leading rounds who were always upbeat, telling patients diagnosed with horrible diseases like cancer, severe heart disease, or chronic obstructive pulmonary disease that they were doing well. None of us were trained on how to deal with death and palliative care at that time. Instead, we were taught multiple ways to treat and perform procedures on patients while they were actively dying.

Despite our encouragement and hopes, Butch's tumor continued to grow, the radiation treatments further inflaming the cancer cells. He couldn't eat and required a feeding tube to supply the little nourishment his diminishing body could absorb, already having lost fifty pounds from his six-foot frame at an alarming rate.

I remember the last time our clinical team rounded on him. We reviewed his tests and lab work from the previous day and answered a few questions. We exchanged light banter, our team again reassuring him, trying to cheer him up before we moved on to our next patient. About ten minutes later, I heard the static clicks of a microphone, the telltale precursor to an announcement over the hospital's public address system. The words that followed were almost always "code blue," an alert that a patient had suffered a cardiac or respiratory arrest somewhere in the hospital. I can still hear the woman's voice that echoed through the hallway:

"Attention: code blue, room 412—Attention: code blue, room 412."

We ran back to his room and found Butch lying on the floor in a large puddle of blood that had formed around his head. Blood poured from his mouth like a wide-open faucet. Two nurses knelt over him, trying to turn him on his side. I stood in the doorway wanting to help and stay out of the way at the same time. My eyes welled up, blurring the rescue measures taking place just a few feet away. I saw images of Butch when we first met; he was chuckling when he asked me to practice my history and physical questions on him, helping pass the time between his different tests and treatments. No one else was crying so I looked away, forcing myself to stop thinking about anything else except this moment, not wanting to appear weak in front of my attendings or chief residents.

It only took a minute or two for Butch to bleed out; a term used by clinicians when a patient loses their entire five liters of red blood cells because of hemorrhagic assault. I learned later that his radiation treatments had eroded one of the large blood vessels in his neck, which carried the majority of blood from his heart to his head.

Butch was my first code blue, and the first time I watched a patient die, learning later in my career that every physician remembers their first patient death. I remembered Butch. He generously allowed me to sit with him for an hour, practicing my interviewing skills taking his history and physical, though he had given it many times before. I spent time getting to know him during our conversations and allowed myself to care about him, something young medical students were cautioned about, unaware of the emotional callouses our tenured residents had firmly in place to protect their psyches.

From 1,300 miles away, I tried not to envision my mother in the final and ugly stages of her disease. Instead, I turned to the coping technique I had perfected over the years: seeking knowledge. Over the next two days, I read everything I could find in medical books and journals on her tumor type, treatment options, and its impact on long-term survival. I was becoming an unlettered neurologist for our family, immersing myself in research on glioblastomas. I sought out top neurologists and neurosurgeons I'd met during medical school or was referred to by others, and asked question after question. The answers only confirmed that Mom's prognosis was not good. Some of the physicians I talked with tried to offer optimistic opinions, but I knew they were trying to cheer me up. A few physicians were brutally honest, telling me that glioblastomas were as bad a cancer as one could get. I appreciated their honesty, developing a stronger bond and trust with those who were open and honest with me.

For the first two months after Mom's diagnosis, I spent hours on airplanes flying to Florida every other weekend while juggling my clinical and learning obligations. Her illness carried into my fourth year of training. On Fridays, I would catch an evening flight, sit at her bedside with my father early Saturday morning in time to discuss her care with her physicians, talk with her nurses before the next shift arrived, and study her chart for any changes. After meeting with Mom's care team, I'd advise my father on the treatment plan that sounded best before flying back to Chicago on Sunday evening in time for early Monday morning clinical rotations at the hospital.

My mother's treatment plan required a craniotomy, a major neurosurgical procedure where they excised a piece of her skull and removed a flap from the top of her brain. Surgery could not remove all of the tumor, so the idea was to remove a large portion of it, referred to as debulking, and then follow the surgery with six weeks of high-dose radiation treatments.

My first weekend trip to Fort Lauderdale was a week after her surgery. Mom had been discharged home from the hospital the day before I arrived and was now aware of her newly diagnosed cancer, the debulking surgery and high-dose steroids having returned her elevated intracranial pressure and level of consciousness to normal. Walking into their apartment and giving my dad a hug, my eyes turned to Mom sitting in a high-backed lime-green armchair in the corner of their living room. Wearing a floral knee-length robe and house slippers, her clothes couldn't hide the swelling in her face, her red, puffy eyes, and her shaved head with three raised incision lines running from one ear to the other. Walking up to her, I gave her a kiss on her cheek and a gentle hug, not wanting to hurt her fragile-looking body. After a weak attempt at a smile, she asked, "How do you like my bald head?" trying to add humor to the emotional moment.

Holding back tears, I replied, "I like the look. Maybe I should shave my head too!" before sitting down on the yellow and lime-green south Florida '80s-style couch next to her chair.

"Your father promised he would buy me a wig. I was thinking of becoming a blonde. What do you think?" Mom's attempts at levity were unable to mask the fear in her puffy eyes of what lay ahead for her.

"Why not go blonde? If you don't like the look, ask Dad to buy you another color!"

Surprisingly, during times she wasn't sleeping, Mom remained in good spirits over the weekend, smiling and putting up a good front. She enjoyed listening to me talk about my different medical rotations, the ones I liked and the ones I didn't like. While it was depressing seeing her like this, we both needed this special time together.

Two weeks later, I was back in Fort Lauderdale. My mother had started her three-days-per-week radiation treatments, permanent blue ink lines crisscrossing her bald head serving as a map for the radiation oncologist about where to aim their radiation guns. Mom was regaining her strength, now able to walk without my dad's assistance, and would always ask about my training, tell me how proud she was, and provide encouragement in ways only a mother can. She was a little forgetful, but happy enough given the circumstances. Unlike her CLL diagnosis, she cast a more upbeat outlook, never bringing up the possibility of dying. Deep down, I knew she was petrified, often gazing out the window, consumed in her own thoughts. We were well aware her time with us was limited, a reality everyone in our family was preparing for in their own way.

After the first couple of months, I traveled to Florida every six weeks and talked with my parents over the phone two or three times a week. Despite the disruption to my personal life and studies, I continued my fourth-year clinical rotations and graduated on time. By late April, Mom's cancer had taken control again and she was too ill to travel, having lost thirty pounds over the last two months. Even on the few good days, she was confused and couldn't ambulate without assistance. Dad, now a full-time caregiver, scheduled a live-in nurse so he could fly to Chicago for my graduation. Mom never watched me put on my long black graduation robe, or step onto the podium to receive my medical diploma. She never heard the dean call me "doctor" as he shook my hand, and she never saw her husband tear up when he congratulated me for both of them.

Dad's presence at the event, seeing the pride in his eyes as he looked up at me on that stage, brought to mind my mother's words of praise years ago on the basement steps, "My David will be a doctor."

After graduation and before my anesthesia internship year began, I flew to Fort Lauderdale to see her. I wanted to show her my diploma and tell her how grateful I was for her love and support. As soon as the cabin door opened, the suffocating south Florida summer air engulfed the entire plane, fogging the windows and my sunglasses. The weight of the humidity caused me to feel faint, and my heart began to beat faster. Beads of perspiration covered the sides of my face and I tasted salt on the edge of my lips. Sitting in an air-conditioned cab, I began to shiver from the dampness of my polo shirt. I felt panicked thinking about how my mother might look, the degree of pain she might be suffering, and how alert she might be during the visit.

When I entered their first-floor apartment, I found Mom in the living room, propped up with pillows in a hospital armchair. My father told me how difficult it had been to rouse her for my visit. His voice broke: "Just getting her out of bed in the morning is difficult. Her pain and depression are getting worse." He didn't need to say anything more. What I saw next was not my mother, but someone close to death. Her condition brought back memories of Butch, my throat cancer patient when our clinical team rounded on him ten minutes before he died. Her face looked translucent with blue and purple veins resembling a road map. Dark circles encompassed her sunken eyes. She weighed no more than eighty pounds and I noted small blisters and sores on her arms. She barely spoke, other than to call out in pain or confusion in a loud voice I didn't recognize.

I remember my father standing next to her, shouting into her ear: "Char, David is here to see you," and "Char, your son is here." Her expression never changed. She continued staring straight ahead, occasionally looking down to pull at her nightgown as if some annoying bug had landed on it. Dad had warned me that I'd see changes in her, but I wasn't prepared for her to treat me like a stranger—to not recognize me. It was painful to feel accomplished as a doctor and yet helpless at the same time. I could do nothing to save my mother.

"Let's get her back to bed," I said as I began to orchestrate the move. I refused to give in to my grief in front of him. I needed to be strong for him.

Her nurse helped us lift her from the chair and set her back in bed.

"I need to take a walk," I told him. Once outside and away from my father, the tears I had held on to for so long were released.

My mother died on a rainy Friday afternoon in mid-September, four months after I graduated from medical school. Earlier that week, I had begun a medical surgical ICU rotation as part of my internship at Michael Reese Hospital in Chicago and had been on call the previous night when my pager went off alerting me I had an outside phone call. Post-call house staff were normally done by noon, but on this day, I was still managing sick patients on little sleep until 3:00pm. Dad was on the other end of the call, and I pressed the phone to my ear wanting to be closer to him. I felt the weight of our loss before he spoke.

"Your mother died peacefully about an hour ago," he said. "She was in no pain as far as we could tell." I remained silent, hanging on to every word. I kept wrapping and unwrapping the phone cord around my chest. "The hospice nurse was with us. The funeral is Monday morning."

His voice broke a few times trying to get this last sentence out. He composed himself and began again. "She suffered far too long."

I still couldn't believe she was really gone.

"How is Debbie doing?" I asked, worried that my sister might have the hardest time accepting her death. From the beginning, Debbie had adjusted easily to her new life in the Sunshine State. But the transition to high school and young adulthood while living as an only child with a chronically ill mother left her struggling to find her place in the world.

"As good as can be expected," Dad said. "She's on her way over now."

"I'll get to Florida as soon as I can. I'm sure my instructors will understand." The silence on the line told me he was trying to wrap his mind and heart around life without his wife of almost forty years. "I love you, Dad."

I didn't cry when I heard the news that day. The reality of her impending death had hit me months before when I saw her for the last time. During my short medical career to date, I had already seen too many patients suffering and dying since I had watched Butch's life end early in my third year of medical school. Like most residents, I had now become emotionally numb to death and was mentally prepared for Mom's death. I needed to be strong for my father and sister, remaining stoic to the pain inside. There would be no more hugs, comforting smiles, or medical questions. My mom was at peace now.

Four years after my mother's death, I was in Fort Lauderdale visiting my dad from the Chicago suburbs where I now lived with my young family. He and I were sitting around his dining room table having one of our regular Friday evening Shabbat martinis together, an old ritual we resurrected after Mom died.

That night he was preoccupied and looked sullen. I feared it might be something health related.

"Dad, is anything wrong? You seem distant."

"I have something to share with you, and hope you don't get upset," he said. I stayed quiet, my concerns about his health elevating. "I shared this with your sister yesterday and asked her not to say anything until I could talk with you today. I need to let you know that you were adopted. Your Uncle Phil was able to work through his network to get both you and Debbie. Your mom and I wanted children more than anything."

His words were thick with apology, though he never said "I'm sorry." I could tell he had weighed his decision to tell us this for some time. He searched my eyes, waiting for a reaction. I smiled, relieved it wasn't his health, and watched a look of surprise wash over his face.

"Dad," I said gently, "I've known I was adopted for a long time. I'm not naïve. There were so many indications through the years. But when I read mom's medical record during her leukemia work-up, any doubts I had were confirmed."

The air in the room lightened. With one of our heaviest family secrets in the open, we both breathed relief. It was a release I had not expected—an important lesson about the weight of secrets.

"I've been wanting to tell you and Debbie for a while," his voice growing stronger in the absence of any anger. "I needed to let you both know that Mom's genes for illness weren't passed down to either of you. You don't have to worry that your children might inherit the same suffering."

When he finished, I rose from the table and hugged him.

"You and Mom are my parents," I said. "I couldn't have had a better childhood." We went back to our martinis, and the smile I had come to love returned to his face.

Through the years, I have learned that every family has secrets. Ours were no better or worse, simply different. But I have also learned that collateral damage created by secrets, deceptions, and lack of open and honest conversations, like the coverups that are perpetuated in health care when patients are harmed, cause lasting physical, emotional, and spiritual suffering.

"Medicine used to be simple, ineffective, and relatively safe. It is
now complex, effective, and potentially dangerous."

Sir Cyril Chantler

On November 29th, 1999, patient safety finally became front page news.
Preventable medical death from errors received national attention when the
Institute of Medicine (IOM) released their landmark report, *To Err is Human:
Building a Safer Health System*. IOM experts estimated that as many as 98,000
people died each year from medical errors in U.S. hospitals.[1] We now know
that statistic was much higher. The report failed to cover the number of
patients who died from medical errors in ambulatory surgery centers and
clinics, or through retail pharmacy medication errors. *To Err is Human* asserts
that the problem is not bad people in healthcare—it's good people working
in bad systems that need to be made safer. And here we are, 23 years later,
addressing the same problem with much higher casualties.

In 2003, author and patient advocate Rosemary Gibson, published
*Wall of Silence: The Untold Story of the Medical Mistakes That Kill and Injure
Millions of Americans.* In the book, Gibson shares personal stories of patients
and family members who had endured medical harm and how they were
treated by hospitals and care teams after these tragic but preventable events.
The book highlighted the fact that most hospitals discourage patients from
gaining access to their medical records, refuse to communicate with families
and, in many cases, flat-out lie to them while attempting to protect the
hospital and healthcare workers from a medical malpractice lawsuit.

---

[1] L.T. Kohn, J. Corrigan, J., and M.S. Donaldson. *To Err is Human: Building a Safer Health
System.* (Washington, DC: National Academy Press, 2000).

This legal strategy, known as "delay, deny, and defend," intentionally delays responses to inquiries about the error, then denies any wrong doings, and defends the care in court with high-priced, high-powered attorneys. When hospitals put up this "wall of silence," the only recourse patients and families have is to seek legal counsel and fight to gain access to the truth. Medical malpractice cases can take years to resolve—that is if the case ever goes to trial. Out of frustration, wanting to move on, or because of a lack of financial resources, many families give up, a strategy hospitals and legal counsel count on.

Gibson's research found that patients and families seek four things after preventable harm: (1) the truth about what happened; (2) an apology, if appropriate; (3) a remedy and resolution; and (4) an understanding on what the hospital is going to do to ensure future patients are not harmed in a similar fashion. The book highlighted the power of three words: *I am sorry*. A simple apology has the power to heal, not just for the patient and family, but for all involved in the medical error, including the healthcare professional(s) who unintentionally harm a patient. Her book helped me envision medical care through an exciting new lens—care that should have been open and honest with James Wilson, our wrong-sided hernia repair patient.

In 2011, David Claussen, MD and colleagues published their research in *Health Affairs*, concluding the use of the "Global Trigger Tool, a series of clues used to identify adverse events at specific health care facilities, demonstrated that preventable medical errors in hospitals may be ten times greater than previously measured."[2]

Data released in 2016 and published in the *British Journal of Medicine (BMJ)* concluded that an estimated 251,000 U.S. patients die in hospitals each year because of medical error.[3] A quarter million patients receiving treatment for chronic conditions like diabetes or having routine procedures like colonoscopies, scans, and biopsies die annually because they experience a medical error during their care. The estimated number of deaths in the *BMJ* study made preventable medical harm the third leading cause of death in the United States behind cancer and heart disease.

A common analogy used to give these hospital death rates context is to compare healthcare to aviation, another high-risk industry. The 251,000

[2] https://www.healthaffairs.org/doi/10.1377/hlthaff.2011.0190
[3] Makary MA, Daniel M.BMJ. 2016 May 3;353:i2139. doi: 10.1136/bmj.i2139

annual deaths from medical error equals 687 preventable deaths each day in U.S. hospitals, the equivalent of four 737-MAX9 airplane crashes every 24 hours, each airplane holding approximately 170 people. Four plane crashes per day in healthcare. The aviation industry stopped all 737-MAX9 airplanes from flying because of two plane crashes over six months. We allow four airplane crashes per day in healthcare and few, including congressional leadership and federal agencies, are aware of or seem to care about these staggering numbers.

Fast forward to February 2020. My own frustrations and feelings of helplessness were overwhelming, not only from the fear of an upcoming pandemic, but from thirty years of working to decrease medical harm with limited success. I, like others, had given hundreds of patient safety presentations at medical meetings around the world, talks that had little, if any, impact on solving the problem. The outcome data on preventable deaths in hospitals was worsening, not improving. I knew, as a physician and patient safety advocate, an additional crisis was brewing. COVID-19 had the potential to increase hospital admissions, deaths, and the number of medically harmed patients. The virus added an additional strain on our already failing healthcare system.

This had been my life's work. I needed to figure out a plan, so outrageous it might add a new urgency to this decades-long problem—something so crazy, it would attract media attention, raise public awareness, and improve patient outcomes.

I kept thinking about Einstein's phrase, "The definition of insanity is doing the same thing over and over but expecting different results." How was I going to stop the repetitious and ineffective strategies that continued to plague our medical system?

The combination of my Friday evening Shabbat martini, followed by a glass of red cabernet, and the viewing of a favorite movie, *Forrest Gump*, gave me hope. My wife and I had both seen the movie several times, but that evening I found my favorite scenes exceptionally poignant. I couldn't stop laughing when Forrest, playing for the University of Alabama, ran the kickoff back for a touchdown and continued running right through the end zone and out the stadium tunnel.

"Must you laugh so loud?" my wife Cathy shouted.

When Forrest innocently lowered his trousers during the White House Medal of Honor ceremony to show President Johnson where he had been shot in the buttocks, my laughter once again earned an annoyed sneer from my wife.

When we reached the scene where Forrest rose from his couch and started running cross country, I leaned closer and watched him run clear to the Pacific Ocean, then turn around and head back. Complete strangers ran with him, asking why he was running. Was there a cause? A mission? The media became interested and started covering his run. Forrest ran coast to coast for over three years before stopping one day, turning to tell the crowd, "I'm pretty tired."

Could I emulate this dramatic scene to alert media and public attention to the tragic safety failures of our healthcare system? I no longer paid attention to the movie, and instead started to play out scenarios in my mind. My running days were over, but I could walk from one coast to the other. This was a totally different approach, a little unorthodox, and admittedly, downright crazy. A sixty-seven-year-old physician walking across America to keep healthcare safety on the radar of colleagues, patients, families, and policymakers.

I grabbed the remote, paused the movie, then shouted to my wife: "I'm going to walk across the country to raise awareness for patient safety!"

Eyes wide, she stared at me like I had indeed lost my mind and then burst out laughing.

"You are crazy!" she said. "Or you definitely had too much to drink. Will you please start the movie so we can keep watching?"

She was getting a kick out of my animation, me being a pretty steady, even-keeled person by nature.

"Tomorrow morning you'll wake up with a headache, regain your senses, and realize how crazy that sounds … especially for someone your age."

We finished watching the movie, but I couldn't stop thinking about this idea that was gaining momentum in my mind. That night, I laid in bed waiting for sleep to come, my brain too activated to fall asleep. Maybe it was a crazy idea. Maybe the martini and the wine made me believe I could do it. In addition to my age, another issue that casted doubt over whether this goal was within reach was my health. During a three-week period in December of 2018, I had been diagnosed with two cancers: thyroid and prostate. Both appeared to have been caught in the early stages, but in 2019 I had two surgeries and radiation treatments and was still recovering. My life now involved follow-up scans, bloodwork, and an arm's length list of diagnostic tests to track if either cancer had spread. I was far from ready to give in to my age; after all, there was still work to do. The question was, could this be the professional home run I had been searching for?

When I woke the next morning, the first thing I did was open my laptop and click on Google. I needed to figure out how many miles it would take to walk across America. The only thing I knew is that I wanted to start with my toes in the Pacific Ocean and finish with my toes in the Atlantic.

"The death of a child is considered the single worst stressor a person can go through."

Professor Deborah Carr
Boston University

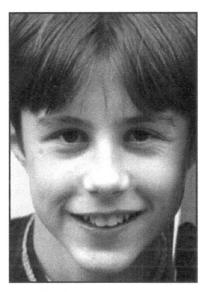

Lewis Blackman
Photo courtesy of Helen Haskell

"It is OK. I come to all the code blues," the pastor said softly, seeing the panic written across Helen Haskell's face. Helen and her husband Bar were standing bewildered and frightened in the hall outside their son Lewis's hospital room, where a crowd of people were surging around his small still figure in the bed.

It is early Monday afternoon. Lewis Blackman, a fifteen-year-old young man, had entered the hospital four days earlier for elective surgery. In medical terms, Lewis had pectus excavatum, a congenital malformation of the sternum, where the breastbone is sunken into the chest. In severe cases, it can compromise a person's cardiac or respiratory function, but that was not the issue with Lewis: his surgery was for cosmetic reasons.

Lewis was an easy-going young man who loved music, especially the Dave Matthews Band. He was a gifted student, active in sports, and his dry sense of humor brought laughter to both young and old.

On Friday, February 26th, 2020, I flew to San Diego to attend the Accreditation Council for Graduate Medical Education's (ACGME) annual meeting where I sit on the Advisory Board for the Clinical Learning Environment Review program. We are tasked with providing U.S. teaching hospitals, medical centers, and health systems feedback on patient safety and quality healthcare education for 140,000 medical residents across the United States. I planned to begin my walk across America on Saturday by walking seven miles along the San Diego Bay harbor. My end destination would be Petco Park, home of the San Diego Padres, and the first of thirty Major League ballparks I planned to visit over the next twelve months. I would begin my 2,452-mile journey across the country by dipping my toes in the Pacific Ocean for good luck, and if all went as designed, I would finish in Jacksonville Beach, Florida, a year later with my toes in the Atlantic Ocean.

For three decades, I had stood behind podiums across the U.S. and around the world as a keynote speaker, addressing audiences at hundreds of healthcare meetings regarding the need to improve healthcare safety. It was clear PowerPoint slides and my passion, along with that of my colleagues, who were also proponents of the need to improve healthcare safety, were not enough to convey the urgency of the problem. Walking off the plane in San Diego that day, I recommitted to this unconventional approach, hoping that, like Forrest Gump, I would inspire others to join me, hoping to bring attention to the story of Lewis Blackman and too many others like him who die needlessly each year, and to the need for change.

For thirty hours over the weekend, Helen had pleaded with hospital staff telling them repeatedly something was not right with Lewis. He had been complaining since Sunday morning about excruciating abdominal pain, a pain much different in intensity and location than the incision pain Lewis was experiencing on *Thursday* evening and Friday after his surgery.

Hospitals can be dangerous places over a weekend, and this weekend the primary physician taking care of Lewis from Saturday evening until Monday morning was an exhausted intern who had begun her pediatric rotation less than a week earlier. When a mother tells you something is not right with their child, you listen and take the concern seriously. Unfortunately, Helen's concerns were brushed off repeatedly. The only other doctor to see Lewis as he declined on Sunday was a senior resident who came from outside the hospital in response to Helen's insistence on an upper-level physician. Without looking too closely, the resident affirmed the nurses' assessment of constipation.

Early Sunday morning, I exited the back door of the Marriott Hotel and found a walkway down to the harbor boardwalk. Walking north along the harbor, I slowed my pace while admiring the variety of sailboats tucked into their slips. Smaller twenty-five-foot ketches, larger two-hulled catamarans ready for charter trips, and each seventy-five-foot monohull racing sailboat favored by professionals in the America's Cup was identified by its unique name painted on its stern. One boat called *Eye Land Dreamer* caught my attention, and I wondered if she might be owned by an ophthalmologist and Jimmy Buffett fan.

On the high-rent side of the harbor opposite the marina stood expansive properties owned by Hyatt, Sheraton, and Hilton. Boaters and tourists eager to spend the day on the water had begun emerging from their hotels, coffees in hand, crowding the walkway. Crew members were readying the boats for excursions, working on decks, loading food and beverages for trips to what I imagined might be Catalina Island nearby. The strong ocean breeze that had forced me to turn the bill of my Cubs cap backwards indicated that today would be a good day to be sailing too. Getting caught up in the nautical spirit of the morning, I picked up a charter pamphlet and thought about looking into a sunset cruise later in the day.

Two miles into the walk, I came upon the *USS Midway* aircraft carrier docked on the harbor side of the boardwalk. Two retired fighter jets sat idle upon its top deck. The powerful steel-hulled ship dwarfed the fiberglass sail and power boats passing behind it in the harbor. Continuing north, I walked by Waterfront Park and stopped to watch children splash in the fountains. Their laughter and giggles while dodging the stream of cool water in the crisp morning air were uplifting, their carefree energy contagious. They would be the first of many people—young and old—whom I would pass along my cross-country route, and who would leave an imprint on my heart and soul.

Reaching the main entrance to the San Diego International Airport, I stopped a third time to admire the commercial airplanes on final approach descending over the city's skyline. Each plane appeared to be less than a hundred feet above the rooftops of the downtown high-rises, yet they landed safely on the ground. It was not a secret that if healthcare could find a way to adopt the same tenets of high reliability that commercial flying had, I would not need to be walking.

Looping back on Harbor Drive through the historic Gaslamp Quarter, the Victorian and Art Deco–style buildings reminded me of the older neighborhoods on the west side of Chicago where I had spent most of my career in anesthesia. From fine dining and steak houses to dive bars and live music, the Quarter had something for everyone. The musty smell of spilled beer hung heavy in the air, and I imagined the late-night party crowd, whose footsteps I now followed, making their way back to home or hotels only hours earlier.

My excitement mounted as I headed inland and saw Petco Park a few blocks away, finally coming to Tony Gwynn Drive, which runs along the south and west sides of the ballpark, and Trevor Hoffman Way that borders the south and east sides. Both streets were named after San Diego Padre Hall of Famers I watched play in the 1980s and '90s. Just walking around the ballpark was energizing, and I unconsciously picked up my pace thinking about the Cubs home opener I would attend in Chicago only a month away. Once again, my thoughts drifted to Lewis....

Just past noon on Monday, an ashen and dehydrated Lewis Blackman lying in his hospital bed turned to his mother and whispered:

"It's ... getting ... dark."

At the head of Lewis's bed, trying to change his pillow, Helen froze in fear. She strained to hear as Lewis repeated himself.

"It's ... getting ... dark."

Before she could react, Lewis lost consciousness, his head and body in full seizure.

Running into the hallway, Helen screamed for help. The resident arrived. Ten minutes later a code blue was called, and an army of physicians, nurses, and pharmacists began streaming into Lewis's room.

An hour and a half later, Helen and Bar were ushered into a small room where a group of five attending physicians were waiting to tell them that their fifteen-year-old son had died. Earlier that morning, medical residents had downplayed the family's concerns. Now the doctors shared that Lewis had died, but they did not know why.

Before leaving Petco Park, I pulled a freshly painted fire-engine-red memorial stone, the size of a small baseball, from my pocket. I had been gathering stones on desert trails during my walks in Arizona after Cathy suggested I find a way to honor those lost to preventable medical harm at each ballpark I walked to. The stone today, which I placed in a small flower garden outside the ballpark, had the name "Lewis" written on it in black ink, in honor of Lewis Blackman. The fifteen-year-old athlete, actor, gifted student, and all-around kind-hearted young man had entered a teaching hospital on a Thursday for elective surgery. He died four days later because of numerous medical errors including failure to diagnose, failure to rescue, misuse of medications, and lack of resident supervision. His mother, Helen, an anthropology doctoral candidate at the time of her son's death, became a staunch patient safety advocate after Lewis died.

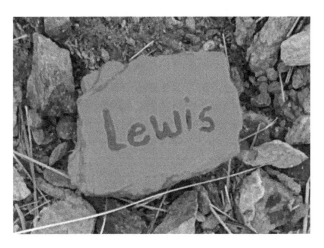

Helen shared some thoughts about Lewis with me:

My son Lewis was fifteen when we took him to a large teaching hospital for an elective surgery that had been highly promoted as minimally invasive and safe.

From the moment we walked into the hospital, we were surrounded by chaos. Within four days, that chaos had cost our son his life. Inappropriately prescribed medication and reluctance to adjust fluid imbalances led to a perforated ulcer. Poorly prepared and unsupervised young weekend staff were unable to recognize a clinical emergency and afraid to call for backup. When Lewis went into cardiac arrest, no one who was present could rescue him. The casualness with which his young life was brought to an end was breathtaking.

It has been many years now since Lewis left us, but the events of those four days are never far from my mind. Our son was one of the top students in our state. He was brilliant, capable, insightful, and intuitively compassionate. People tell us they are sorry for "our" loss, but that is taking the narrow view. The loss is to us all. What might he have become? What would he have given back? The unnecessary loss of thousands of souls a year has unfathomable implications for every one of us. We can never measure the distance between what is and what might have been.

All the metaphors you hear about losing a child are true. When Lewis died, it was like a part of me had been torn out. He was my lifework. When he was little, our bedtime reading was an atlas. I would tell him as much as I knew about all the places in the world that he could someday visit. My biggest regrets are all the things he never got to do. He never fell in love and he never traveled, the thing he wanted most in the world. I had filled him with a yearning to see the world but in the end he never even rode on an airplane.

Since Lewis died, the world has changed in ways I would never have predicted—although Lewis, a modern teenager with his finger on the pulse of the dawning century, might have made some good guesses. In health care, however, too much remains unchanged. I was propelled into patient advocacy when I realized that the dysfunction I had witnessed in Lewis's care was not unusual; his care-givers had, in fact, been following standard processes for an American teaching hospital. In our case, as in many others, the luck on which the system relied simply ran out. Even now, after years of patient safety reforms, I continue to hear stories like Lewis's. Yet the solutions—training, technology, teamwork, attention to the patient—seem basic and commonsensical. What will it take to motivate change if patient deaths are not enough?

In academic medical centers, most attending physicians trust patient care to house staff—residents and interns on call overnight and on weekends—who at times can be taking care of forty patients or more. While an attending physician is a phone call away, many residents fear calling their attending in the middle of the night. The adage "Calling an attending is a sign of weakness" is heard often, the expectation being that residents should figure the problem out themselves.

Lack of adequate resident supervision happens far too often today and at times can lead to serious preventable patient harm or death. As Helen shared with me, the primary physician taking care of Lewis for most of the weekend was a single exhausted intern who had begun her pediatric rotation less than a week earlier.

Every resident physician remembers at least one "night of terror" related to the lack of attending supervision. Mine came at the end of my second year of anesthesia residency. Finishing the last of three emergency surgeries, I headed to my call room around 2:00am, hoping to get a couple of hours sleep. Laying my head on the plastic pillow, my pager started beeping, the flashing phone number alerting me to call the intensive care unit. John Piano, the fourth-year surgical resident on the other end of the phone, rapidly recited a brief history of a critically ill eighty-year-old man who needed an emergency cystoscopy to remove a kidney stone that was obstructing urine flow from his right kidney, causing a severe pyelonephritis infection. The elderly man was in the early stages of septic shock, his blood pressure low and heart rate high.

Calling my anesthesiology attending who was sleeping comfortably in his warm private call room, I let him know about the emergency case coming to the operating room. He told me to get the operating set up and he would be down shortly.

Dr. Piano transported our critically ill patient to the operating room where I quickly reviewed the patient's medical record. Approaching the transport bed, I stuck out my hand and introduced myself.

"Mr. Sandoval, my name is Dr. Mayer, I am the anesthesia resident who will be taking care of you tonight. Dr. Monroe, my attending, will be here shortly."

Eugene Sandoval said nothing, continuing to moan in pain, barely conscious from his bloodstream infection and looking sicker than the surgical resident had described over the phone twenty minutes earlier. Mr. Sandoval's breathing was rapid and labored, his respiratory muscles weakening with each gasping breath. His mucous membranes were dry from dehydration and his skin was cold and clammy—more warning signs of impending septic shock.

After moving Mr. Sandoval to the operating room table and quickly placing all my monitors, it was time to put him asleep but my anesthesia attending was nowhere to be found. The surgical team and nursing staff were staring a hole through me, anxiously waiting to get started. Mr. Sandoval's condition was worsening with each minute. His only chance was to remove the kidney stone and hope the antibiotics would take care of his infection and sepsis. I had put patients to sleep before without an attending in the operating room—heck, in a year I would be finished with my residency and be doing this by myself every day. But I was scared. Mr. Sandoval was extremely sick and I wanted twenty years of experience standing behind me if something went wrong. Hoping Dr. Monroe would walk through the operating room door shortly, I nervously administered the anesthetic induction medications, the needle twice missing the IV administration port because of my trembling hands.

After successfully placing the breathing tube in the patient's trachea, I proceeded as trained, connecting the tube to the ventilator circuit and taping it in place. I then watched in horror as my patient's systolic blood pressure took a serious drop: 100 ... then 80 ... then 60 ... then 50. Was Mr. Sandoval dying in front of me? I knew septic patients could have serious blood pressure declines right after they are put to sleep, but I'd never witnessed such a rapid decline like this. I tried to get the nurse's attention, hoping she could find Dr. Monroe, but everybody was frantically busy doing their work as I struggled to keep my patient alive.

The next thirty minutes became a reflexive balancing act, administering different vasoactive medications alternating between small doses of epinephrine and Neo-Synephrine to raise Mr. Sandoval's blood pressure to a normal range without causing it to spike so high that he would incur a stroke or heart attack. I had never worked that hard during a surgical case, mentally or physically, over a thirty-minute period in my young career, perspiration now soaking the upper half of my scrub shirt. Charting the patient's vital signs during the surgery was impossible; he was so unstable that I never had even ten seconds to relax and catch my breath. I had been in such a stressful "zone," doing everything I could to keep my patient alive, that it wasn't until the surgery was over and we returned Mr. Sandoval to the intensive care unit that I realized my attending had never shown up.

At 7:00am, I found Dr. Monroe in the break room drinking coffee and looking well rested. I hadn't slept all night, my nerves still buzzing from the intensity of the last few hours. He apologized, saying he fell back to sleep right after I called. He had awakened a couple of hours later and called the operating room. When a nurse told him the case was over and that the patient was back in the ICU, he hung up the phone and went back to sleep. Seeing him well rested and cavalier about the surgery made me furious inside, but I bit my lip and remained silent.

Mr. Sandoval was critically ill and difficult to manage for a seasoned physician. Both the patient and I needed Dr. Monroe's knowledge and experience that night. It was only by the grace of God that my medically fragile patient was returned to the intensive care unit alive.

"Every nurse was drawn to nursing because
of a desire to care, to serve, or to help."

Christina Feist-Heilmeier

Two days after beginning my walk across America in San Diego, the Patient Safety Movement Foundation's (PSMF) Board Chairman and Founder, Joe Kiani, called an emergency board meeting. I had recently been chosen to replace Kiani as CEO of the PSMF and had sat on the organization's board since 2013. Rumblings of what would soon be labeled the SARS2-CoV-2 virus was taking hold in China and Europe, and conditions were shaping into what might soon become a global pandemic. The PSMF Annual Summit was scheduled to start that Thursday, March 5th in Irvine, California, and attendees from Taiwan and Japan had already cancelled their trips because of safety concerns in China and the Pacific Rim.

Because our guest list included President Bill Clinton as a keynote speaker, along with hundreds of patient-safety leaders from around the world, the safety of our attendees was the primary topic on our agenda. It soon became clear to all of us who worked in health care that this virus was more contagious, and therefore more dangerous, than anything we had experienced in our lifetimes. And while the monetary impact of cancelling with only three days' notice to the hotel, the caterers, and our entertainment would be substantial, our board unanimously decided to do just that because of safety concerns. The PSMF would be one of the first major medical meetings to cancel its spring gatherings. We were all a little unnerved by the number of infections being reported early on, so instead of heading directly back to the MedStar Health corporate office in Maryland, I decided to fly to Phoenix on Wednesday afternoon and work from my home office until we had more information.

MedStar Health, the largest mid-Atlantic ten-hospital health system where I serve as executive director of the MedStar Institute for Quality and

Safety (MIQS), was beginning to see patients arrive in their emergency rooms in respiratory crisis in unprecedented numbers. New York City had been hit hard early on and many hospitals in the northeast region of the country were soon overrun with patients gasping for air, their oxygen saturation plummeting, causing a shortage of available ICU beds and ventilators. In just a few days, it was clear that patient and healthcare worker safety initiatives would take a backseat to the public health crisis emerging around the world. This, in addition to the growing impact of the virus on our most vulnerable patient populations in our biggest cities, concerned me the most.

The following week businesses began to shut down, work-from-home orders were issued by Fortune 500 companies, and many non-essential workers around the country were let go, furloughed, or headed for a stressful year of uncertain employment. The sports world followed in step. On March 11th, 2020, the National Basketball Association (NBA) suspended its season until further notice. On March 12th, the National Hockey League shut down play until it was "appropriate and prudent to continue." On the same day, Major League Baseball (MLB) halted the remainder of all spring training games and postponed the start of the regular season for two weeks. And, on March 13th, the NCAA March Madness men's and women's basketball tournaments were cancelled. Ballparks and stadiums across the U.S. went silent and the nation held its collective breath awaiting the next panic-laden newscast. On March 16th, Major League Baseball announced that the start of the 2020 season would now be pushed back even further, at least until late May.

The country was now officially locked down, something none of us had ever experienced in our lifetimes. We cancelled spring break family vacations with our kids and grandchildren, and I worried about when I would be able to next see them. Would we be locked down for six weeks? Six months? A year? Would this pandemic follow a similar course as the Spanish flu pandemic did in 1918, taking two years of our lives? It was depressing to spend too much time thinking about the what-ifs. When MedStar Health issued "work-from-home" orders for all non-essential personnel, it meant I was going to be sequestered with Cathy at home in Arizona until further notice. I worried about how I would continue to collaborate with my team back in Maryland who all were also confined to their homes. I worried about the medical and nursing students and resident physicians who were now facing the most challenging training conditions in over a century.

On the morning of Sunday, March 29th, I was sitting on the couch after an eight-mile morning walk when Cathy's voice jarred me from a moment of post-walk relaxation.

"Can you please get off my couch with that wet shirt. Your perspiration will make the couch smell!" She sounded near horrified as she came into the room. "And how many times have I asked you to take your dirty running shoes off in the garage before you come into the house. Who knows what you stepped on out there!"

My wife is a germ freak. I used to tease her when we were younger, but I have learned over time how right she has been. After once watching a mother change her baby's diaper on top of the seatback tray on an airplane, I soon switched to her camp on high-alert mountain, noting that not everyone felt the same need to keep the environment contagion-free.

I jumped up and headed to the garage where I removed my running shoes and tossed them by the side door to air out. When I walked back in the house, it was as if she had continued the conversation without me.

"I'm very concerned about your walk across the country." A retired shock trauma and neurosurgical ICU nurse, she understood the risks viruses pose to those with comorbid conditions, like cancer, and who were already immuno-compromised like me. "The early data is showing people over sixty-five are at high risk of dying if they get infected. Plus, you just finished treatments for two different cancers, which adds even more risk for you."

I listened more intently now, her love and concern coming alive the more she put words to her fears. She could not help but have noticed the urgency emanating from our MedStar Health system updates being held three times a week. The patients continued to flow into our emergency rooms, validating the severity of this virus in real-time. With 10 hospitals and 280 non-acute centers, our health system was able to respond in ways New York City hospitals could not. We could move physicians and nurses around when and where it was necessary. We also had the space and transport services to move patients, both affected and unaffected by COVID-19, to both control the infection and address the volume of health-related demands of the Washington DC, Baltimore, and Maryland areas we served. The virus was proving to have a regional virulence, some even referring to it as the Amtrak virus because of infections being higher along the work-related train routes in the corridor between Baltimore, Washington DC, Newark, New York, Connecticut, and Boston. South of Washington DC in Virginia, up in Maine and across the plains and western states, people were questioning the truths coming out daily on the evening news. For those in the northeast, it could not have been more real.

"Maybe you should hold off until we see how this evolves. Why not do the walk next year when baseball season resumes, and the stadiums will be open to fans?"

"Who knows what next year will bring?" I calmly replied. "My arthritic knees are not getting any younger. I do not want to wait until next year. Plus, if history repeats itself, this pandemic will be with us for at least two years. Next year will be just as dangerous."

"Patients are continuing to die. And now our colleagues at the front lines are also dying because we were not prepared for this pandemic. I cannot sit at home and do nothing."

By the look on Cathy's face, she knew what my answer would be before she asked the question, but she had to share her fears. She does not like to admit it, but Cathy is also over sixty-five years old and at a higher risk if we proceeded. Caregivers by nature and profession, we were both having a tough time sitting on the sidelines and needed to feel like we were doing something.

"I completely understand but needed to put the question out there for discussion. Your mission and commitment to do this walk and our colleagues at risk at the frontlines outweigh our own personal risks."

After a short pause, she added, "But we need to do everything humanly possible to keep ourselves safe."

All too soon, news reports began honoring healthcare professionals from all areas of acute-care facilities who became infected and died while doing what they loved—taking care of patients. We watched regular news footage of New York and Washington DC police and firefighters who parked outside hospitals, all standing to applaud patients and healthcare professionals struggling inside. *Kaiser Health News* almost immediately partnered with *The Guardian* to host a series called "Lost on the Frontlines," which posted stories of the heroism performed by nurses, doctors, first responders, and ancillary healthcare workers who fell victim to COVID-19. Both Cathy and I became regular readers of the series, wanting to understand the lived experiences of our colleagues, and learn more about how this virus was behaving. Two of those stories especially caught my attention. The first was about a physician at an inner city New York hospital:

Dr. J. Ronald Verrier, a surgeon at St. Barnabas Hospital in the Bronx, spent the final weeks of his audacious, unfinished life tending to a torrent of patients inflicted with COVID-19. He died April 8th at Mount Sinai South Nassau Hospital in Oceanside, New York, at age 59, after falling ill from the novel coronavirus. Verrier led the charge even as the financially strapped St. Barnabas Hospital struggled to find masks and gowns to protect its workers—many nurses continue to make cloth masks—and makeshift morgues in the parking lot held patients who had died.[4]

The second was about a nurse who worked at a Veterans Affairs hospital:

Nurse Vianna Thompson, 52, spent two nightshifts caring for a fellow Veterans Affairs health care worker who was dying from COVID-19. Two weeks later, she too was lying in a hospital intensive care unit, with a co-worker holding her hand as she died. Thompson and the man she treated were among three VA healthcare workers in Reno, Nevada, to die in two weeks from complications of the novel coronavirus. Thompson, who dreamed of teaching nursing one day, died April 7, joining a growing list of health care professionals killed in the pandemic.[5]

What began as a crazy idea suddenly also became a way to honor others during the most uncertain time in our lives. Nurses, physicians, and first responders were putting themselves in harm's way without adequate protective gear and proper training to safely treat the rapidly escalating number of patients. These were colleagues and friends, resident physicians, and nursing students who had attended my Academy for Emerging Leaders in Patient Safety Summer Camps over the last ten years running straight into the fire this virus had created. They were working long shifts and then staying overnight in hotels to isolate themselves from family members, fearful they might bring the still-evolving virus into their homes. They watched in horror as their morgues quickly filled, leaving nowhere to put the dead. These were our heroes, putting patients first while also risking their lives without the proper protection. If they had to show up during the pandemic, somehow so did I. They could not quit; I could not quit either. I had to keep walking.

---

[4] "Lost on the Frontline". KHN.org. Kaiser Health News and The Guardian. August 10, 2020.
[5] "Lost on the Frontline". KHN.org. Kaiser Health News and The Guardian. August 10, 2020.

Since I could not change what was going on in the world, I forced myself to look at the positives in my immediate environment. Being locked down in Arizona in March had its advantages. I was not in New York, Maryland, Washington DC, or anywhere else in the northeast part of the country where the virus was now rampant. Not to mention, March weather in Arizona is as good as it gets. The cool, dry mornings and moderate sunny days with temperatures in the seventies and eighties were made for outdoor activities like hiking, biking, and walking. I forced myself to focus on the things I could control.

Nonetheless, I was taking extra precautions to stay safe while walking. With infection and death rates climbing exponentially in many parts of the country, it would only be a matter of time before the virus made its way to the southwest. Social distancing soon became everyday language and I made certain to distance myself from others on the paths and sidewalks. When indoors shopping for groceries, I wore a surgical mask and a plastic face shield.

News programs hungry for the facts and latest stories covered COVID-19 twenty-four hours a day. They reported on what we knew and speculated on what we did not know. Depending on the political spin of the channel, those truths could be vastly different, fueling mistrust over the true death and infection rates. It was when the news coverage began pulling in stories from front-line healthcare workers that only those blinded by political ideology could fail to see we were being tested like never before. Reporters put their own lives in jeopardy to interview ICU nurses, many through tears when reliving the loss of up to ten patients in one eight-hour shift, watching them drown on dry land, unable to breathe because of the virus's grip on the respiratory system. Only weeks into the pandemic, nurses were voicing exhaustion and how burned out they were. Those inclined to depression were quickly overwhelmed, while even those with the most stable mental health were pushed to the edge.

Inner city communities, people of color, and the elderly trapped in long-term care facilities and their caregivers were being hit hardest in February and March before we had a handle on how to manage the virus. None of this should have been surprising for anyone paying attention to the minefield that is public health. The longstanding mistrust of our healthcare system held by Black and Brown families because of our failure to address decades of health inequities and the silver tsunami already poised to take down our skilled nursing facilities were gaps that should have been addressed decades earlier. The magnitude of the lives lost early on, like that of preventable medical harm, might have been curtailed if hospitals had safety and quality processes hardwired into their systems. Instead, we watched just short of helpless as the virus devastated families who lost loved ones in our hospitals and nursing homes, unable to provide comfort or say goodbye at the bedside. More than ever, I knew I had to continue forward with my walk across America to remember not only patients who died needlessly from preventable harm, but also caregivers who were dying because of our inability to have properly planned for a pandemic so many warned would eventually come. The truth is that working in health care has never been a safe occupation. Workplace injuries, depression, burnout, and suicide rates are higher than in most other industries including construction, and only now is legislation being enacted to protect our healthcare professionals. Still, the aftermath of caring for patients through a pandemic has forever changed our workforce.

During one of my morning walks in mid-April, an idea hit me while listening to "Go Cubs Go" by Steve Goodman on my iPhone. The song is played after a Cubs win at Wrigley Field, and fans sing along not yet ready to let go of the energy in the park. Arizona has one Major League Baseball team, the Diamondbacks who play at Chase Field, but the area has ten spring training facilities spread throughout the Phoenix Valley. Many of those ballparks are shared by two Major League teams, which made for fourteen different MLB teams in state. I decided to stay local and walk to all ten spring training parks, testing the environment locally—in the waterless desert—before embarking upon a cross-country road trip. I would begin at Sloan Park, home to the Chicago Cubs, walk to the remaining nine Cactus League ballparks and Chase Field, and then finish back at Sloan Park.

Once home, I began mapping out different routes on my computer. I would have to walk 125 miles over ten days to make this happen, a few of the days requiring about fifteen miles between two of the ballparks. My longest walk up to now had been about ten miles, so I would need to increase my daily mileage over the next few weeks to be ready for those longer distances. I could feel my excitement returning now that I was finding a way to bring baseball stadiums back into my walk across America, despite the ballparks being closed.

What I did not consider in my deep desire to keep moving forward was that late May temperatures in Phoenix regularly hit the upper nineties, often hitting triple digits. The dry heat would add another level of difficulty to an already outrageous goal. Nervousness began to creep in. I wondered if my passion for righting these long overdue wrongs had finally taken hold of my common sense.

"You treat a disease, you win, you lose. You treat a person,
I guarantee you, you'll win, no matter what the outcome."

Patch Adams

Friday, May 22nd, 2020

Total miles walked since February 28th, 2020 = 614
Total steps taken = 1,605,434

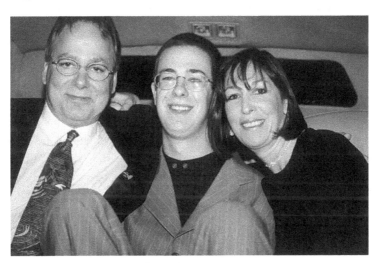

David, Michael, and Patty Skolnik (1996)
Photo courtesy of Patty Skolnik

*Inquiring about the neurosurgeon who would be operating on their twenty-two-
year-old son in two days, hospital staffers assured Patty and David Skolnik of his
skills, one even commenting:*

"He is the best neurosurgeon in the hospital!"

It was not until later after Michael was lying in a coma that they discovered he was the only neurosurgeon in the hospital.

I could not think of a better place than Sloan Park, the spring training facility of the Chicago Cubs, to start my 125-mile walk across the Phoenix Valley. Three months to the day, on February 22nd, 2020, Cathy and I had been sitting twelve rows up from the Cubs dugout under a cloudless blue sky, watching the Cubbies pound the Oakland Athletics 12–2 in the spring training opener. Four days later we were back at the ballpark watching the Cubs defeat the Kansas City Royals 8–0, the saguaro-lined Superstition Mountains providing an artistic backdrop behind the right field fence. This was my definition of relaxation, and with two solid spring training wins on the books, the 2020 season looked promising for my hometown favorite. The thought that those two games would be the last I would attend in 2020 never entered my mind.

Rumblings of a pandemic-strength virus discovered in Wuhan, China, had only begun to materialize in the U.S., but they quickly shifted to a thundering reality when our day-to-day life came to a halt in mid-March. The pandemic not only stopped baseball, America's greatest pastime, it also closed basketball and hockey mid-season. At the same time, it changed the way we worked, played, and loved. All too close to home, it presented the greatest test to our national healthcare system, our medical supply chain, and to generations of nurses, physicians, and first responders in over a century.

Baseball had always been there for me—a way to unwind and let the stress of caring for babies born prematurely with congenital heart disease or end-stage pulmonary patients struggling to breathe while waiting for a double-lung transplant fade into the cheers of Cubs fans surrounding me in the "Friendly Confines" of Wrigley Field at the corner of Clark and Addison on Chicago's North Side. Without the comforting din of a ballgame on television in the background, or the full sensory overload of sitting in the bleachers at Wrigley, I was without a go-to coping mechanism when COVID-19 patients began to fill the intensive care units and morgues in hospitals across the country. I hoped that my ten-day walk across the Phoenix Valley to all ten Cactus League baseball parks would quell my anxiety and fill an existing chasm in my life. I could not wait to begin.

Michael Skolnik's strength was his gentleness; his weakness was trying to help save everyone including a three-legged cat and many others from the animal kingdom.

His devotion to helping others was why he chose to enter the nursing profession. Suffering from a new onset seizure, a CT scan revealed a three-millimeter spot on the top of Michael's brain. The neurosurgeon told the Skolniks that Michael needed urgent surgery to remove what he believed was a possible small pineal cyst. It would be a simple 1.5-hour procedure because the cyst was easily reachable sitting directly on top of his brain. Without the urgent surgery, however, Michael might die.

Before I went to bed that night, I positioned twelve bottles of water, six bottles of Gatorade, and six bottles of Vitamin Water in the front of the refrigerator, ready to grab in the morning. My wife, Cathy, our sag wagon driver and part-time walker, had prepared individually wrapped peanut butter and jelly sandwiches, fruit, nuts, and protein bars. The empty cooler was loaded in the back of the car, with bags of ice in the freezer, ready to be added in the morning.

In just two short months of lockdown, the pandemic was becoming a dangerous football for political pundits, and the rhetoric was playing out in strange ways across Arizona, a purple state still trying to figure out if the pandemic was real or a hoax. We were uncertain how people from both sides of this growing, volatile argument would perceive our mission while walking through some of the richest and poorest communities in the Phoenix Valley. Because of my training as a physician and Cathy's training as a trauma and critical-care nurse, we respected the work virology and infectious disease experts were reporting as they sorted through the data and evolutionary nature of COVID-19. This virus scared us because it was so contagious and was taking lives faster than experts could find ways to stop its progression. We planned to wear the masks that were becoming more a political statement than an adherence to a simple public health solution. These were the same masks I wore every day in the operating room for over twenty-five years without hesitation to protect my patients from infection.

Before getting into bed that evening, I gathered the clothes I strategically planned to wear the next morning. The spring desert required layering to meet the extreme shifts in temperature from early morning to midday. The dry earth, clumps of dirt and rock, and roadside route demanded our legs and eyes be protected. I began placing my favorite, well-worn pieces on the guest room bed: lightweight, black running pants; a bright-colored T-shirt to keep me visible while walking along the roadside; my grey, sweat-stained Maui North Beach baseball cap worn since starting my walk across America;

cushioned-heel Thorlos ankle socks; and black-and-blue Brooks Glycerin running shoes. When I placed the last items on the bed, I felt a presence behind me. Cathy was standing in the doorway with a smirk on her face.

"How long have you been standing there?" I asked.

"Long enough to know you're a little obsessive, maybe borderline pathologic," she said.

"How long have you known me?" I asked, seeing the humor in what she might perceive as eccentric behavior. "There is always a method to my madness. I do not change a routine that works. Do you want to see me running around in a panic trying to find one of my Thorlos in the morning?"

She turned to get ready for bed leaving me to my pre-walk ritual without saying anything. Then she could not help herself. "Maybe you should just get dressed tonight and sleep in your outfit!" she shouted over her shoulder.

I paused, briefly considered her suggestion, and then moved on to my final task for the evening, which was to ceremoniously pull out my vintage 1953 Chicago Cubs jersey. It was one of twelve Cubs jerseys hanging in a special section of our bedroom closet, all neatly pressed and aligned like a visitor might observe in a Cooperstown Hall of Fame display. Earlier in the week, I had put considerable thought into choosing this jersey. It was my favorite because 1953 was Ernie Banks's rookie season with the Cubs, and it was also the year I was born. The cream-colored, wool jersey had the classic Cubs logo on the front right side and the number 14 on the back. Like all uniforms from that era, only the player's number was on the back of the jersey. On May 22nd, 2020, I would be wearing the number made famous by Mr. Cub, also the first number to be retired by the Chicago Cubs in 1982. Each day of my walk, I would choose a different Cubs jersey, all having sentimental value marking the decades of my Chicago sports fandom.

Diehard Chicago Cubs fans understand that there is a cadence and an intentional, annual commitment in rooting for the Cubs. Before manager Joe Maddon arrived in 2015, we watched teams from New York, St. Louis, Oakland, Philadelphia, and Kansas City celebrate October baseball and playoffs over 120 times, our season mathematically over long before the final games were played in late fall. Cubs fans have endured the longest off-season for decades, except for the rare occurrence when the Cubs made the playoffs only to lose in the first round. Our season did not begin again until late February with the start of spring training, roughly 140 days after the Cubs last game of the year in early October. The Cubs had played 113 seasons, making the playoffs just fourteen times. If you throw out the 1907 and 1908 seasons when they had last won the World Series, the Cubs won just one playoff series in 106 years.

In 2003, for the first time in fourteen years, the Cubs earned the title of National League Division series champions after beating the Atlanta Braves three games to two. They then advanced to the infamous National League Championship Series against the Florida Marlins. With the Cubs leading the series 3–2, they held a convincing 3–0 game and series winning lead going into the top of the eighth inning. Every fan in Wrigley Field could taste a shot at the World Series. Generations of Cubs fans sat in expensive, ticket-brokered seats dressed in winter coats, protecting themselves from the fifteen-mile-an-hour winds and deceiving 50-degree nighttime temperatures that dropped with each gust of wind. Thousands, if not millions, of fans sat glued to their televisions, ready to break open champagne in tandem with the team. However, an avid Cubs fan became a household name in Chicago after accidentally interfering in Moises Alou's attempt at a foul ball in the left field box seats. The meltdown on the field that followed resulted in eight runs scored by the Marlins, and another loss in the final game of the series the following day.

Being a Cubs fan was almost genetic, the allegiance passed down from one generation to the next despite the curse. "Wait until next year," had been a well-known refrain spoken by Cubs fans, including me, until 2016 when the faithful were rewarded with the Cubs' first World Series championship in 108 years. For those who bleed Cubby blue, those losing years shaped our collective character, forcing loyalty, eternal hope, and a short memory for the team's failures. Next season held every opportunity for success and we waited for the fun to begin all over again. I could not wait for the following season's schedule to be released and would immediately circle two dates on my winter calendar: the day pitchers and catchers reported to spring training, and the spring training home opener in Mesa, Arizona. It did not matter to me that the star ballplayers only played an inning or two that first day, hitting the showers early to get in eighteen holes at a local golf course. Sitting in the bright Arizona sunshine watching baseball in February was a break from Chicago's harsh winter and a pleasant reminder that spring and opening day at Wrigley Field was only six weeks away.

Michael Skolnik's surgery lasted six hours. No cyst was ever found and Michael suffered permanent brain damage from the operation. His health continued to worsen while suffering multiple infections and breakdowns in care, dying thirty-two months later due to the medical errors. Although Michael's surgeon claimed to have done this specific surgery numerous times, it was later discovered that he had only performed this surgery once before.

Four days before the start of my Arizona walk, Lisa Riegle, our good friend and neighbor, heard about my ten-day walk across the Phoenix Valley and asked if she could join me, eager to support our patient-safety mission. Her good friend Barbara Black also asked to join us. We welcomed them, grateful for the company.

We arrived at Sloan Park at 4:30am, an hour before sunrise. Standing at the front gate of the park, I pulled an orange-painted stone from my pocket, the name "Michael" written on it in black ink. Michael Skolnik was taken to the operating room for an unnecessary neurosurgical procedure and died thirty-two months later at twenty-five because of multiple medical errors starting with an incorrect diagnosis, followed by preventable complications and hospital-acquired infections that occurred during and after his surgery. Michael's mother, Patty Skolnik, walked away from a successful career to become an advocate for safer care. Her passion and commitment to patient safety and shared decision making led to the Michael Skolnik Medical Transparency Act passed in 2007 by Colorado legislatures.

Patty shared this passage about Michael with me:

Our Michael was twenty-two when a neurosurgeon performed unnecessary brain surgery and destroyed his life. Michael suffered horrendous preventable harm, the operative word being preventable, for thirty-two months before he died. He was courageous, a fighter, empathetic and touched the hearts of everyone that met him. These are some quotes from those that knew him.

"Patricia, I am writing you to let you how much your son meant to me and our friends. Michael was three years older than me but still took me in, fed me, and gave me a place to live. It brings tears to my eyes to know that this Earth is short such a dynamic person. Mike would take me to school and always made sure I went. He was wild and crazy at times and had a tremendous sense of humor. My success in life would not be what it is if I had not had your son's leadership and knowledge. I just wanted to let you know that your son has touched so many people with his compassion, wisdom, and his reach for the stars." Drew

"I am at a loss to understand why one family and one young man who did nothing to deserve any of this would have to suffer so. Michael deserved to have a long, full life and it is not right that he will not have that and that you will not be able to share that life with him. I hope you find comfort in knowing that Michael knew more clearly than most are able to know how very much his parents loved him and would give your all to him. I instantly connected with Michael the first time I met him. He was so engaging! Bright, full of life, interesting, fun, funny, and an independent spirit. His message to all of us is that life is short and precious and, because you never know when it will be taken from you, live. I hope we can take a moment together to toast Michael and raise our glasses to what a special person he was and how he lit up the lives of so many people." Mary

Michael was our heart and there will forever be a huge hole that cannot be filled. Not an hour goes by without a thought of him. We miss him no less and even maybe more seventeen years later.

The health system was broken then and unfortunately as hard as we try there is still much work to be done to fix it.

I cannot think of a worst trauma than losing a child. I have a friend who lost a child who says, "I'm constantly wondering where he is. Where he has gone. It's like a wheel turning at the back of my mind. He can't have just vanished. He must be somewhere."

Michael Skolnik—and Lewis Blackman whom I remembered at Petco Park in San Diego—are two of 250,000 people who die needlessly each year. Every one of these deaths ripples out into families who are forever changed. With Lewis and Michael's deaths, parents lose a child, siblings lose a brother or sister, and grandparents lose the precious moments and memories a grandchild can bring them. The senseless loss of these two young men had solidified my movement into patient safety leadership and were representative of the reason I was walking across America. After laying the stone in a small garden just outside the ballpark, I led a short memorial service for Michael, recounting stories Patty and David had told me about their son. We then stood in a moment of silence to honor Michael and his parents.

"The single greatest impediment to error prevention in the medical industry is that we punish people for making mistakes."

Dr. Lucian Leape

We left Sloan Park and headed east, the sun still beneath the Superstition Mountains in front of us. I had carefully mapped out the day's 14.4-mile walk using Google Maps and kept track of our progress on my Fitbit. Fifteen minutes into our walk, a young calf approached the chain-link metal fence that bordered the one-acre property, a single-story wooden house sitting in the back of the lot. The calf eyed us with warm curiosity, pushing its nose through an opening in the chain-link fence trying to sniff us out. This was the first of many inquisitive onlookers we would meet along the way. The young calf allowed us to pet him, earning him the name "Norman" after Billy Crystal's affectionate calf in the movie *City Slickers*. We all agreed it was a positive omen to start the day.

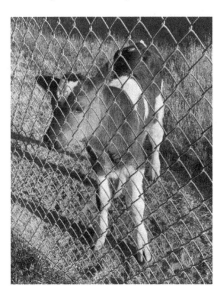

An hour into the walk, the metal tower stadium lights rising above the tree line were a telltale sign we would soon be arriving at the new Hohokam Stadium, currently the spring training home of the Oakland Athletics and former home to the Cubs from 1997 to 2013. The Cubs played at the original Hohokam Stadium from 1979 to 1996, named after the Hohokam people believed to have lived in the Mesa, Arizona, area from AD 1 to the 15th century. Thanks to the loyalty of Cubs fans and the harsh Chicago winters driving sun-seeking spring break escapes, the team consistently broke attendance records, and our family contributed to those numbers. Before making Arizona our second home in 2009, Cathy and I packed up the kids along with swimsuits, sunscreen, and Cubs caps, T-shirts, and jerseys annually, spring baseball being a great reason to flee the frigid Chicago Februarys and watch Sammy Sosa, Kerry Woods, Mark Prior, Aramis Ramirez, and manager Dusty Baker prepare for the upcoming season.

I had not been to Hohokam since 2013 and wanted to take time to explore the now green-walled, yellow-trimmed ballpark decorated with life-size pictures of the Oakland A's star pitcher Chris Bassitt and first baseman Matt Olson painted on the walls. I walked alone around the perimeter of the park and imagined the game that should be going on beyond the walls. I closed my eyes and pictured the parking lot full of cars and buses, the crowd roaring with each base hit, and the familiar call of hot dog and beer vendors. For a moment, I forgot about the intensity of 2020.

Walking past the center field gate, I came upon an elderly man who looked to be in his eighties. He was also enjoying a morning walk in the safety of the parking lot. On top of his head was a tattered green and yellow Oakland A's baseball cap protecting his balding head from the morning sun. He greeted me with a nod and pointed to my jersey. We stopped to chat from a safe distance since both of us were in considerable risk if we contracted the virus.

"This is A's territory now," he said with a laugh, his eyes smiling above his mask.

I laughed. "What gets you up this early in the morning to walk around an empty baseball stadium?"

He pointed to an older, three-story red-brick condominium building across the street. "I am retired and have been living in that building for almost twenty years. This is my regular route. Helps me stay young. What gives with the old-school Cubs jersey? And what are you doing up so early, walking around my ballpark?"

I told him about my plan of walking to all ten spring training ballparks over the next ten days to raise awareness about patient and healthcare worker safety.

"You're crazier than I am," he said, echoing Cathy's initial reaction. "Have to love your passion for baseball though. I can relate. Hope you make it to all of them."

We continued to chat about our love for former baseball greats Reggie Jackson, the A's Hall of Famer known as Mr. October for his World Series heroics that helped the A's win three straight World Series championships from 1972–1974, and Ernie Banks, the Cubs Hall of Famer who never played in a single post-season game. If the pandemic had not stopped baseball, I would have purchased two grandstand tickets and invited him to join me. I was enjoying our banter and would have liked to extend the moment between two old baseball fans sharing trivia and reliving memories that brought to life so much more than baseball—a game that once again proved to be a way of making friends out of strangers.

When our group left Hohokam Stadium en route to Salt River Fields, a ballpark shared by the Arizona Diamondbacks and Colorado Rockies, we had 11.3 miles yet to cover. Miles seven through twelve proved to be the most taxing ground covered since I began walking over two months earlier in San Diego. From Mesa to Scottsdale, we were on a four-lane road without sidewalks, forcing us to traverse vacant fields through knee-high grass and weeds. The road had been torn up, expanded to meet the traffic demands of Maricopa County, the fastest-growing county in the United States. Locals attributed the growth to Californians cashing in on inflated home prices and escaping the highest tax rates in the country. In the Phoenix Valley, they had greater purchasing power and could own less expensive, larger pieces of real estate with much lower property taxes.

We waved at construction workers laying down new pavement in the growing morning heat, their faces covered in dirt and sweat. Dump trucks and pavers driving back and forth forced us onto the shoulder, and we were directed to cross uneven, dirt roads numerous times to keep from being run over by one of the fast-moving heavy vehicles kicking up chunks of the dry desert. My new running shoes were now covered in dirt and matched my black walking pants, also coated with a layer of thick, gray dust. Lisa, Barbara, and Cathy had paid an unforeseen price for choosing to walk in shorts, their legs blending into the grayish-black earth from the knees down. Our sunglasses protected our eyes from the dirt and small rocks, but we could not avoid the pebbles pelting our exposed skin while we were walking down the road. We thought we had planned for everything but walking through a construction site tested our collective endurance.

Halfway through the construction area, we passed a large cigarette store. It was the first building we had passed since leaving Mesa about an hour earlier, the ten-foot-tall sign in the parking lot an eye-catching advertisement for the 360 flavors of cigarettes sold inside. The single-story building looked to be fifty years old and needed a new coat of paint. The windows and entrance were protected by steel security gates. Because of pandemic restrictions, customers were not allowed inside to purchase cigarettes and were instead sitting in cars waiting to access the single drive-up window on the side of the building. I counted over forty cars with even more people inside them waiting to stock up and feed their nicotine addictions despite the road construction, traffic delays, and pandemic risks. Suddenly all the enlarged hearts and blackened lungs I had witnessed in operating rooms made sense, reinforcing how strong behavioral choices drive the overall health of our society.

We arrived at Salt Rivers Field just after 12:00pm where a FOX TV cameraman was waiting for us in the parking lot. His camera may have captured our physical exhaustion as we approached the front gate of the ballpark but seeing him provided the surge of adrenaline I needed to forget about my aching knees and burning feet. Settling in for the interview, I was able to let go of my discomfort and refocus on the mission.

"How long have you been a Chicago Cubs fan?" asked the reporter.

"All my life! I am walking 125 miles across the Phoenix Valley over ten days in memory of the 250,000 patients who die each year due to preventable medical harm, and all the healthcare workers who are dying needlessly because of the pandemic."

"How many ballparks are you walking to?" he asked.

"All ten Cactus League ballparks and then Chase Field to raise awareness of how often medical errors occur," I said. "Your viewers likely have no idea this is the third leading cause of death in the U.S."

Each time he asked me about baseball or the desert heat, I acknowledged his question and then turned to the problem of preventable medical harm and the toll the pandemic was taking on our healthcare workforce. I thanked him for coming out to cover my walk, and when we finished only then did exhaustion take hold. I could not wait to get home, shower off the layers of desert and let the water cool my sunburned face. The next item on the day's agenda would be a short nap to recharge for our Friday evening Shabbat celebration with our son, Scott, and his family over FaceTime.

In the Jewish religion the Sabbath, or Shabbat in Hebrew, begins Friday evening at sunset. Biblical stories describe the creation of the Heaven and Earth in six days, with Shabbat marking a day of rest that occurred on the seventh day of the week, which for Jews is Saturday. Because days in the Jewish calendar start at sunset and finish the following sunset, Shabbat starts at sunset on Friday evenings and is reserved for spending time and sharing festive meals with family and friends.

Despite my parents' traditional Jewish practice, we celebrated an abbreviated Shabbat. On Thursday evenings after dinner, my mother was in the kitchen making gefilte fish, which in Yiddish means "stuffed fish," and chicken soup for Friday's festive meal. Like her mother and generations of Jewish mothers before them, she used her mother's wooden chopping bowl and metal grinder to chop up deboned whitefish, carp, and pike. She mixed in breadcrumbs and egg to keep the baseball-sized fish balls she rolled by hand in one piece.

Her chopping bowl once belonged to Bubby Cupcake. It was a well-loved family heirloom at least forty years old with a chunk of wood missing at the top. One year, while visiting from college, I bought my mom a new chopping bowl for Mother's Day.

"I love it," she said after unwrapping the present. She walked over and gave me a kiss on the cheek. The gentle smile on her face told me there was something more she wanted to say. After a thoughtful pause, she continued.

"The bowl is such a thoughtful gift, and I can understand why you chose it. Would you be upset if I return it?"

"Not at all," I said, confused. Her old bowl had seen better days.

"Every week, when I pull that bowl out of the cabinet, it reminds me of Bubby Cupcake. It is as though she is in the room mixing gefilte fish with me."

I nodded, understanding well the need to keep Bubby Cupcake close. Mom was helping me see what I would soon come to realize: that material things matter far less than the history they hold.

On Friday evenings we gathered as a family for dinner. The familiar ritual of watching my mother light the Shabbat candles minutes before sunset and shortly before my father came through the back door was grounding.

Dad would stop to give us all a kiss before heading upstairs to clean up before preparing his weekly martini. In addition to his family, my father had three loves in his life: collecting stamps, playing chess, and his regular Friday evening martini. He always started the Shabbat weekend with a gin martini before sitting down to our family's festive meal. Outside of weddings and bar mitzvahs, Friday night was the only night I ever saw my father drink alcohol.

Unlike James Bond's Vesper martini made of three ounces gin, one ounce vodka, and one-half ounce of dry vermouth, my dad's martini was straight Beefeater gin with a wave of vermouth. I enjoyed watching the care he took preparing his cocktail. The small, waist-high wooden liquor cabinet in our dining room held the ingredients, and he worked like a chemist in the laboratory, measuring and mixing the precise amounts of reactants to produce the desired product. With a smile on his face, he poured exactly three ounces of gin into his 1940s glass shaker followed by a single drop of dry vermouth, claiming it was the single drop that made his martini extra dry. Next, he added exactly four ice cubes before carefully securing the steel lid so that he could shake the mixture until the ice broke into small crystals. Once satisfied, he unscrewed the dime-sized cap covering the pour spout and filled his favorite long-stem martini glass, the ice crystals floating around three green olives he had prepared on a plastic toothpick resting at the bottom of the glass.

When I turned sixteen, my dad let me taste his martini for the first time. I raised the martini glass to my nose, smelling his drink and feeling grown up. The first thing that came to mind was kerosene. I took a tentative sip that only confirmed gin was a match for his palate and not mine. I disliked the taste even more than the smell but did not want to spoil the rite-of-passage moment with my dad by complaining.

Once Dad finished mixing his martini, we would sit in our usual spots around the dining room table and watch while my dad placed his skullcap, known as a yarmulke in Yiddish and a kippah in Hebrew, on his head. My mother always made sure to place it on his dinner plate when she set the table each Friday afternoon.

My father began our Shabbat meal using our family's abbreviated version of the customary service. He only knew how to sing two prayers in Hebrew, the blessing over the wine and the blessing over the challah, so that was the extent of our festive meal service. The Kiddish, or the blessing over wine, sanctifies the day of Shabbat and recognizes its holiness. When he started the blessing, we would all join in:

בָּרוּךְ אַתָּה יְיָ אֱלֹהֵינוּ מֶלֶךְ הָעוֹלָם, בּוֹרֵא פְּרִי הַגָּפֶן.

We would then recite the English translation together: "Blessed are You, the Lord our God, King of the Universe, Creator of the fruit of the vine."

After the prayer over the wine, my father removed the white cloth that covered the golden-brown braided challah my mother bought each week at the Skokie Bakery, which was the place to be on Friday mornings with hundreds of Jewish women from surrounding suburbs lining up to purchase the cherished loaf of bread. We would next recite the blessing over the challah:

בָּרוּךְ אַתָּה ה' אֱלֹהֵינוּ מֶלֶךְ הָעוֹלָם הַמּוֹצִיא לֶחֶם מִן הָאָרֶץ

And then we followed with the English version: "Blessed are You, the Lord our God, King of the Universe, who creates bread from the earth."

After prayers, we enjoyed the challah, gefilte fish with deep red horseradish, and homemade chicken soup. All were favorites of mine, and I always asked for seconds. This not only pleased my mother, but it also filled me up so I could avoid eating the main meal my father chose every week: boiled cow's tongue. This was an Eastern European dish his mother made when he was young, and to say I hated it is an understatement. I would have drunk Dad's entire gin martini if it meant I did not have to eat tongue. The football-sized, flesh-colored cow's tongue sitting in the middle of a large platter surrounded by boiled cabbage leaves looked like something straight out of a horror film. The blood vessels and tendons on the pharyngeal portion of the tongue where it had been sliced from the cow's throat were still visible at one end, the little round papillae, or small bumps, visible on the tip of the tongue at the other end of the organ. The sight of it made my stomach clench and was immediately followed by a wave of nausea. My mother forcing me to eat it was like a scene from a bad commercial. Our dog, a white toy poodle named Zipper, learned to sit under my chair and enjoyed as much of my main course as I could sneak under the table.

Years later, when my father passed away, I came across his old glass cocktail shaker while packing up his possessions. The shaker now sits in my liquor cabinet, and I use it every Friday to make my Shabbat martini. My routine is without the same fanfare as my father's, but I always think of him when I mix my Hangar One vodka martini with a splash of Cointreau, the hint of orange reminding me of a sandy beach on a tropical Jimmy Buffett-like Caribbean island paradise. My son Scott and I have continued my father's Friday evening ritual of celebrating the end of the work week and coming of Shabbat with a vodka martini toast over FaceTime as often as we can. Once my son and I have caught up on highlights from our work week, Cathy and our daughter-in-law, Leah, often join with a glass of wine. Our two grandchildren, Brody and Joelle, wait with excitement for airtime with Grandpa and Gigi, Cathy's grandmother moniker.

After we returned home from our first day of walking through Phoenix, this comforting Shabbat ritual brought my parents into the room with us. I especially missed them at times like this and hoped that they were looking down with pride from above. My time with both seemed exceedingly short and being unable to share my success and mission with them left an ache in my heart that evening. Like Cathy and the elderly Oakland A's fan I met earlier in the day, they would have thought I was crazy, but I am certain they would have been proud of my life's work.

I logged onto FaceTime with martini in hand and connected with Scott to toast the day's accomplishment and the Shabbat. I thought about Lewis Blackman and his mother, Helen. I thought about Michael Skolnik and his mother, Patty. I pictured the empty seats at their dinner tables during family celebrations like Shabbat. I looked into my son's eyes across the digital miles and thanked God that I could share this moment with him. Silently, I recommitted to my walk across America no matter the physical or logistical challenges we might face in exchange for the hope that someday no parent would have to experience the grief Helen, Patty, and too many parents like them carry every day for the rest of their lives.

Before going to bed, I watched the *FOX News* interview from earlier in the day. The segment was only ninety seconds, but my plan had worked. Those watching *FOX News* that evening heard about a sixty-seven-year-old doctor walking in the Arizona heat, asking colleagues and patients across the country to join him in raising awareness of the need to improve patient and healthcare worker safety. I went to bed hopeful, thinking that walking across America during a lockdown was not such a crazy idea if I could help save lives.

"It is not the things we get, but the hearts we touch that will measure our success in life."

Charlie Brown (Charles M. Schultz)

Saturday, May 23rd, 2020 (Day Two of the Arizona Walk)

The sound of my alarm chirping on the nightstand about two feet from my head at 3:30am woke me from a deep sleep. Day two's walk would be fifteen miles, starting at Salt River Fields with a stop at Scottsdale Stadium, the home of the San Francisco Giants, before finishing at Tempe Diablo Stadium, home of the Los Angeles Angels.

The decision to wear my Joe Maddon jersey that day was easy. Maddon was the manager who led the Cubs to their first World Series championship in 108 years. Back in 1961 and 1962 when Philip K. Wrigley owned the ball club, the Cubs used a "College of Coaches" model instead of one traditional manager like other teams, four coaches rotating as head coach for parts of the season. The experiment failed miserably, and the Cubs moved back to one head coach from 1963 to 1965 but continued to lose ball games. In 1966, the Cubs hired the fiery, in your face, "Nice Guys Finish Last" Leo Durocher to manage the ball club. Durocher, known as "Leo the Lip" because of his constant arguing with umpires from the dugout, had previously managed the Brooklyn Dodgers and New York Giants. He loved kicking dirt on umpire's shoes while screaming at them in disagreement with one of their calls. Because of his antics on the field plus his accused association with gamblers off the field, Durocher was suspended from baseball in 1947. He returned in 1948, being named manager of the New York Giants. leading them to a World Series championship in 1954. Leaving the Giants after the 1955 season, he became a TV color commentator until 1966 when the Cubs named him manager.

Durocher's tenure as manager didn't last long, as he got fired midway through the 1972 season. The Cubs used twenty-six different managers over the next 43 years before hiring Joe Maddon to manage in 2015. Maddon was the opposite of Leo Durocher, a calm, soft-spoken manager liked by players, fans, and the media. Before coming to Chicago, Maddon managed the Tampa Bay Rays between 2006 and 2014, twice being named MLB Manager of the Year. You might disagree with his baseball strategy or tactics at times, but everyone respected his knowledge and love of the game. Maddon did unusual things that kept his players loose during the long 162-game season. One year he organized a petting zoo on the Wrigley Field outfield grass for players, coaches, and their families. The zoo animals included a snow leopard, sloth, penguin, armadillo, and pink flamingo. He brought the pink flamingo to his pre-game media session, talking to reporters with the flamingo sitting on his lap. On one red-eye plane flight back from the Cubs west coast trip, he made his players and coaches wear bright-colored children's-style pajamas (one-zees) and gave awards to players with the best-looking pajamas. He had a list of sayings, many ending up on T-shirts, things like "Try Not to Suck!" and "Respect 90", (the ninety-foot distance between bases), wanting his players to always hustle. His passion for the game of baseball was palpable. In 2019, with the club looking like they would be going through a rebuild, Maddon left Chicago and was immediately hired to manage the Los Angeles Angels.

Lisa, Barbara, Cathy, and I were back at Salt Rivers Park around 5:15am. Before beginning our walk, I pulled a bright yellow memorial rock with the name "Josie" printed on it in black letters from my pocket. I laid the rock on a small patch of grass outside the stadium while sharing Josie's story with our group.

Josie King was an eighteen-month-old brown-eyed, light-brown-haired child who loved to dance. She had just learned how to bounce on the trampoline with her siblings and how to say "I love you." She was admitted to a hospital after suffering first- and second-degree burns climbing into a hot bath. Josie healed well, but two days before discharge, she died from dehydration and mistakes made in administering a narcotic pain medicine. Her mother Sorrel used the personal tragedy to start the Josie King Foundation. The foundation's mission is "to prevent patients from dying or being harmed by medical errors" and it provides innovative safety programs and care journals to hospitals and caregivers that help reduce harm at the bedside.

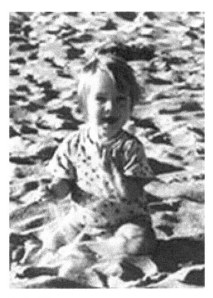

Josie King
Photo courtesy of Sorrel King

Sorrel is an amazing human being and someone I have had the great fortune of calling my friend, supporter, and mentor through the years. She gave me permission to share this paragraph from her own book, *Josie's Story*:

I realized as I flew home that Josie's story had struck a chord with the very people who could fix the problem. I could not stop thinking about their reaction, how they listened to me, how they cried and confided in me. They seemed hungry for something, though I wasn't sure what. Maybe it was the fact that I was coming at patient safety from a different angle. I wasn't talking about the data and statistics. I didn't have a lengthy PowerPoint presentation. I wasn't one of them: I was an outsider with a real story.

After a moment of silence for Josie, we began walking south where we were treated to newly paved sidewalks through upper-middle-class communities. Our route to Tempe Diablo Stadium took us through Historic Old Town Scottsdale. Founded in 1894, the upscale community has an Old West charm, mixing expensive restaurants, hotels, shops, art galleries, and night clubs with Old West blacksmith shops, century-old churches, and historic school buildings. Porsches, Ferraris, and Mercedes lined many of the streets. Residents were out walking, running, or biking on Saturday morning wanting to beat the midday heat. Only a small number were wearing face masks, as if the pandemic had miraculously missed the rich, affluent community of Scottsdale.

Arriving at Tempe Diablo Stadium, we had completed another 16.2 miles over six hours in the ninety- to one-hundred-degree desert heat.

Sunday, May 24th, 2020 (Day 3 of the Arizona Walk)

Starting back at Tempe Diablo Stadium, Sunday's walk would be another sixteen miles. Over the first two or three miles, multi-storied metal and glass Fortune 500 office buildings lined the street, the stately two-story lobbies, glass door entrances, and expansive reception desks ready to greet visitors. At mile three, the neighborhood changed dramatically, with junkyards now taking up real estate along the street. Rusted cars without wheels, dented washing machines, and other metal debris was scattered throughout the properties visible behind eight-foot chain-link metal fences topped with barbed wire to prevent trespassing. If the fence and barbed wire were not enough of a deterrent to unwelcome visitors, "Guard dog on premise" signs were mounted on the fence every ten feet, with angry German shepherds running back and forth, barking as we passed.

Cathy parked our car around mile eight in an older two-story office building parking lot that looked safe and waited for Lisa and me. It being a holiday weekend, the building was closed and the parking lot empty. Ten minutes later, a white Honda Civic turned into the parking lot and pulled up next to Cathy. The middle-aged African American woman who was driving the car rolled her window down. Surprised, Cathy rolled her window down too.

"Are you OK?" the woman asked. "I was out for my morning run and saw you sitting alone in your car. It is not common to see a blonde-haired white woman sitting alone in this neighborhood. I was worried something was wrong. When I finished my run, I jumped in my car and drove back to check on you."

The woman's concern for Cathy's safety offset the worry my wife first felt having a stranger pull up next to her in the empty parking lot.

"That is so nice of you to drive back and check on me," Cathy replied. "How sweet of you to do that. I am fine but thank you. Most people would not do that."

The woman introduced herself as Laria and the two struck up a conversation, my wife telling her why she was parked in the lot and what we were doing. Laria shared that she is a counselor for abused teenage women. Over the course of the next twenty minutes, each learned more details about one another's work and how they were both trying to make the world a better place—Cathy in patient safety and Laria devoting her free time to helping young foster girls find safe homes. Laria shared that her own daughter had been abused by her ex-husband, and she had to fight for two years to gain custody of her daughter after their divorce. Learning how to navigate the legal system, Laria said she found her calling in life by helping other abused young girls find safe homes. After sharing contact information with each other, she drove out of the parking lot and headed home, but she stayed in Cathy's heart. This was the first of so many acts of kindness we would encounter over my walk across America, reaffirming for me during very challenging times that despite all the political polarity, bigotry, antisemitism, and ugliness going on across the country, there are so many wonderful and caring people in the world once we get past our internal bias and open our hearts to each other.

Looking at my Fitbit watch, the white numbers illuminated on the black face let me know we had just passed ten miles for the morning. The high-rise hotels and office buildings of downtown Phoenix pierced the sky about a mile to our north. The massive steel-beamed retractable roof of Chase Field, the home of the Arizona Diamondbacks baseball team, was also visible just south of the metal and glass downtown skyscape. Looking down East Buckeye Road, several large cardboard boxes lying on dirt and rock about ten feet off the sidewalk came into view. We were approaching a homeless village with more than twenty individual cardboard structures scattered across the vacant lot, each consisting of three or four brown boxes cut along the side and taped together with gray duct tape, creating additional space within the four-foot-tall living quarters. A sheet of blue plastic hung over the top of many domiciles, serving as protection against the few drops of rain that might visit the desert valley. About two dozen homeless men and women were sitting on plastic crates in front of the paper abodes. My internal biases had me nervous, moving to the opposite side of the street, trying to keep a safe distance from the tenants of these cardboard homes. I even contemplated turning down a side street to avoid conflict. My own anxiety about what might happen next halted my conversation with Lisa, as I wanted to stay focused on getting us safely past this self-perceived potential trouble spot along our route. This was a different fear, an uncertain fear from what I felt when construction trucks raced by us just ten feet to our side. As we began passing the first cardboard home with its tenants sitting out front, I kept looking forward, hoping not to make eye contact and draw attention to the two strangers in comfortable exercise clothes and running shoes walking past them. Voices began to call out "Good morning," "Nice morning for a walk," and "Where are you two heading?" To my surprise, most were wearing masks and following social distancing, their plastic crate chairs about five or six feet apart from each other. Unlike affluent Scottsdale, the poorest areas in Phoenix seemed to understand there was a killer pandemic going on and were trying to stay safe. Lisa and I slowed our pace, looked across the street, waved, and yelled "Good morning to you too." We smiled, acknowledging it was a nice morning for a walk as we continued walking and waving. Everyone we passed waved to us. By the look in their eyes it was obvious they were smiling under their masks, enjoying the rare occurrence of visitors walking through their cardboard community early on a Sunday morning. As we emerged from the rows of homeless villages and entered downtown Phoenix, I began laughing at myself. Growing up in my sheltered Jewish bubble created fears, many that were unwarranted. The warm welcome we received from the poorest people living on the street in this homeless community was one of the friendliest and uplifting greetings I received over the entire ten days of walking through the Phoenix Valley.

Finally arriving at American Family Fields, our walk turned out to be 17.3 miles. Driving home, the tiredness and quiet we all appreciated in the car had me reflecting about the last three days. The pandemic was making life inconvenient for the rich, many now having to wear masks when in public places, but it was more than just an inconvenience to the poor, bringing high infection and mortality rates to those living on the streets who had little if any access to the healthcare system.

Over the first three days, we had now walked fifty-three miles in the desert heat. The three longest days of walking were over, making me believe Monday's ten-mile walk would be easy.

Monday, May 25th, 2020—Memorial Day (Day 4 of the Arizona Walk)

I found myself wanting to roll over and go back to sleep when wakened at 3:30am. My mind was in a fog, not able to concentrate on the early morning tasks at hand. We had pushed ourselves hard the first three days, walking fifty-three miles in the extreme heat, and I wanted a day off, but it was not going to happen. Lisa was not quitting either, her support helping me push forward.

We drove back to American Family Fields of Phoenix, the spring training site for the Milwaukee Brewers. Before starting our walk, I took a few minutes to enjoy the beauty of the ballpark, coming across six-foot-tall bronze plaques of Milwaukee Hall of Fame ballplayers lining the left and right field sides of the park: Robin Yount ("The Kid"), Hank Aaron ("Hammerin Hank"), and Paul Molitor ("The Ignitor"), to name a few. Coming to the last plaque, I could not help but laugh, my early morning blues quickly vanishing. The plaque honored Bob Eucker ("Mr. Baseball"). A catcher by trade, his fame came in the broadcast booth and he was often touted as one of the best commentators in the game. Appearing frequently on the *Tonight Show* with Johnny Carson, his dead-pan sense of humor was legendary for baseball lovers. Playing Harry Doyle, the radio announcer for the Cleveland Indians in the movie *Major League*, his sarcastic humor helped make the movie a baseball classic.

With my Kris Bryant Cubs jersey on my back that morning, we started heading north to the Peoria Sports Complex, home of the Seattle Mariners and San Diego Padres. Cathy drove our car to mile five where we found her parked on a side street immediately off a major highway. The two-block-long street was dirty, with broken glass bottles and flattened beer cans scattered against the curbs. Numerous cracks and potholes, wider and deeper than those seen in Chicago after frigid winters, had me wondering how Cathy navigated all the bunkers safely. The street was lined with single-story apartment buildings built in the '70s, cracks running in all directions on plastered walls that desperately needed a new coat of paint. The apartments reminded me of the Bates Motel in the Alfred Hitchcock movie thriller *Psycho*. Each apartment building had four small units looking no bigger than a motel room. The front lawns lacked grass—just dirt and rocks with an occasional bent clothesline for drying clothes.

Cathy raised the trunk of the car as we approached, all of us now congregating at the rear of the car pondering what cold fluids we needed from the cooler. After picking up a bottle of Gatorade and turning away from the back of the car, I noticed a middle-aged Hispanic man come out of one of the apartments, cross the street, and walk toward us. He was wearing old grey shorts, a dirty white sleeveless T-shirt that struggled to cover his protruding belly, and faux leather slippers with no backs on them, causing him to shuffle his feet as he approached us. My immediate thought was that he would be telling us we could not park our car in front of his house, my own bias again making me think the worst with a confrontation coming from an angry tenant.

He stopped about twenty feet from us and shouted, "Are you OK?"

Everyone now turned around, hearing the man's voice.

Nervously, I replied "Yes, we are OK," hoping he would turn around and go back into his home.

He started walking toward us again, stopping about ten feet from the back of our car. While not wearing a mask, he appreciated the importance of social distancing.

"That's good to hear," he replied as a big smile came across his face.

"I saw the trunk up and thought your car had broken down. Don't see many people, especially a young blonde woman with a newer Audi, parked on our street." That was the second time we had heard that comment, his words reminding me of the African American woman who came to Cathy's aid in the parking lot on day two.

My nervousness had now evaporated like the sweat on my face and I turned on a big smile myself with his concern about my wife's Audi. You could also tell he had a way of charming people with his comment about "my young blonde" wife. Cathy had made another new friend and we all laughed.

"I am a mechanic and when I see a trunk up, I think flat tire or bad battery issues. Wanted to make sure it wasn't anything like that."

We were all touched and thanked him for his kindness, sharing with him what we were doing and why we were doing it. Like so many others we had met along our way, he laughed aloud and said we were crazy walking in this heat but impressed we would take on such a task to help others.

His voice going up an octave, he excitedly said, "Wait here while I go back inside and get you some cold bottles of water."

We pointed to our stocked cooler and told him we were well supplied. He then had another idea. "You can surely use some cold towels to put on our necks to cool off. Let me go inside and get some."

Cathy stopped him again, sharing that she had thought of that too and cold towels with a bag of ice were also in our cooler.

We could not believe how caring and generous this gentleman was. By all looks, he had little money but was willing to give us bottles of water and cold towels to take with us without hesitancy. After spending another fifteen minutes talking with him, we told him we needed to start walking again so we could finish by late morning. Before we left, he reached into his pocket and handed me one of his business cards.

"If you have any car issues or need help over the next few days, call me. I will drop what I am doing and come help."

Smiling, I replied, "Thank you."

He turned and shuffled back to his apartment.

The immense generosity of this man was another of the many examples of human kindness I experienced during my walk across America. I will always remember his giving personality and still have his business card in case I do need a mechanic in the valley someday.

Finally arriving at the Peoria Sports Complex, Monday's walk turned out to be just short of twelve miles. Despite having three more TV media outlets there at the end to interview me, I was mentally drained and could not wait to head home and take a nap. The fourth day had been the toughest day so far despite the shorter mileage and the wonderful generosity of our new friend.

"A journey of a thousand miles begins with a single step."

Laozi

Tuesday, May 26th, 2020 (Day 5 of the Arizona Walk)

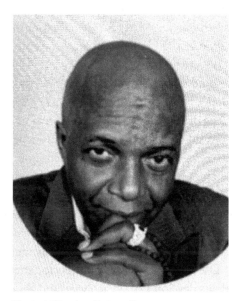

Yogiraj Charles Bates, II
Photo courtesy of Vonda Vaden-Bates

"The doctors are busy saving lives."

This is the response Vonda Vaden-Bates received from hospital administrators when she asked why the doctors who took care of her husband would not meet with her after her husband's death.

Charles "Yogiraj" Bates II was an author, entrepreneur, father, master trainer, sage and fearless advocate for the human spirit who suffered preventable medical harm from a series of misdiagnoses and lapses in standard of care. These errors led to his death while hospitalized from a deep vein thrombosis (DVT) and ultimate pulmonary embolism.

Yogiraj's wife, Vonda Vaden-Bates, asked for subsequent meetings with hospital administrators and the physicians who took care of her husband. Wanting to learn what had happened and have their family's questions answered so she could help others in similar situations, her meeting with administrators was first postponed and then cancelled, and her request to speak to the physicians taking care of her husband received the "too busy saving lives" response from the hospital. When preventable medical harm occurs, many hospitals lock down and turn all communications over to their legal team, denying families answers to their questions.

Day five's walk would take us from the Peoria Sports Complex to Surprise Stadium, spring training home of the Texas Rangers and Kansas City Royals. Vonda Vaden-Bates had driven from California and met us at the Peoria Sports Complex, joining our walk today. In 2020, Vonda drove across the country by herself, and over the course of 129 days she covered more than 10,000 miles and visited thirty-six cities in twenty-nine states. She conducted twenty-seven interviews with patient safety experts which she posted on social media. Vonda walked over 700 miles in support of my walk across America, raising money and awareness on behalf of the Patient Safety Movement Foundation's mission. Vonda lost her husband, Yogiraj Charles Bates II, because of a misdiagnosis after incurring a DVT and preventable blood clot after surgery. Approximately 300,000 patients develop DVTs each year, and about 10 percent result in death. Healthcare has evidence-based prophylaxis protocols that have been shown to significantly reduce deaths from blood clots. The use of compression socks, blood thinners and early ambulation after surgery are among those protocols, but when safety protocols are not followed, people like Yogiraj die.

Since her husband's death, Vonda has dedicated her life to making care safer for others, becoming a national thought leader in the prevention of deep vein thrombosis.

Standing near the home plate entrance to the Peoria Sports Complex, I pulled a green-painted memorial stone with Yogiraj's name printed on it in black ink out of my pocket. I placed the stone on the gravel-covered ground and led another short memorial service and moment of silence in his honor.

Vonda sent me the following passage about her late husband:

The day I met Yogiraj Charles Bates I began to see and learn differently. I think of him as Toto in The Wizard of Oz, *pulling back curtains to reveal what is really happening. He was a master at analyzing movies and fairytales and would most certainly be amused at my analogy. Having lived his life with a knack for compassionately uncovering hidden truths, my beloved husband's death did more of the same. He was hospitalized for thirteen days following a craniotomy to address a subdural hematoma, and several missteps obscured the development of one of the most common ways people die from hospital-associated conditions. A cascade of concealment would only be revealed after his death from a venous thromboembolism (VTE).*

Yogiraj Charles' autopsy would lift the veil on neglect to assess his risk for VTE and prescribe necessary prophylaxis to prevent a well-known, preventable complication following lengthy surgeries. A lack of education and commitment to safety at the hospital resulted in failure to identify my husband's obvious symptoms of both deep vein thrombosis and pulmonary embolism. As a result, he was not diagnosed or treated appropriately. But the most important revelation his death prompted for our family was a deny-and-defend culture in health care that impedes learning and perpetuates errors, harms, and fatalities across the globe every day. The moment our beloved died in that ICU room, he became a risk the administration was managing rather than a patient the clinicians and staff had cared for over thirteen days.

Applying compassionate care while helping people and systems see and intervene upon hard truths was Yogiraj's special gift. My fervent wish is that it will be mine too as I shed light upon the need for, and support interventions necessary to prioritize, the safe delivery and receipt of medical care. The Wizard of Oz intentionally concealed because he did not understand how to accept the limits of his power while also conveying his wisdom. With coaxing from Dorothy and her companions, including Toto, the Wizard learned to find and play to his strengths.

Our way home to the land of 'do no harm' is most certainly in need of a transparent brick road; one that learns from errors—whether harmful or not— and disseminates lessons for the benefit of everyone. May my husband's hospital experience and his legacy of expertise, which he trained hundreds of others to apply, support the road to zero harm.

About an hour into our walk, we passed through Sun City, Arizona, home to a large number of retirement communities and an abundance of different golf cart styles owned by its residents—not the type of golf cart one sees on golf courses, off-white in color with two hard cushion seats and a place on the back for two sets of golf clubs, but customized golf carts painted in every color of the rainbow. The golf carts are approved for street driving, having front head lights, back taillights, racing-style rear-view mirrors on both sides, shiny chrome hub caps on extra-wide tires, and a horn to alert people as they speed past. Some are customized to look like a small Mercedes Benz or Rolls Royce. Retirees use them to shop, dine, or just see how fast they can race with cars on the street, making me wonder whether a few have been nitro-super-charged like drag racers to impress the neighbors.

The last part of our walk was through farmland, making me wish I was walking through the cornfields of Dyersville, Iowa, with Ray Kinsella's *Field of Dreams* ballpark appearing in the distance. Arriving at the ballpark, I was struck by the beauty of Surprise Stadium. A combination of burnt red and light pink cinder blocks circled the park, the stone resembling spiritual red rocks found in Sedona two hours to the north. Looking through the stately white picket fences connecting the stone columns, the deep green manicured grass covering the outfield, the recently groomed brown dirt on the infield, the bright white chalk lines of the baseball paths lining both sides of the diamond made for a picture-perfect moment. The white picket fence railings running along the right and left field upper deck grandstands gave the park a Churchill Downs Racetrack appearance awaiting the annual Kentucky Derby horserace.

Wednesday, May 27th, 2020 (Day 6 of the Arizona Walk)

Day six's walk was from Surprise Stadium, home of the Kansas City Royals to Camelback Ranch-Glendale Stadium, spring training home of the Chicago White Sox and Los Angeles Dodgers. I chose to wear my Ben Zobrist autographed #18 Cubs jersey because Zobrist played for the Royals in 2015 when Kansas City won the World Series, then came to the Cubs in 2016, and proceeded to become the Most Valuable Player in the 2016 World Series, helping bring Cubs fans their first World Series since 1908.

With little to see along the walking route besides open fields and vacant lots, I sought out things to amuse me and started counting small plastic liquor bottles lying on the side of the road, the ones displayed on checkout counters at liquor stores. Our walking group picked up on my suggestion, counting over one hundred small plastic liquor bottles in under two hours, almost half being New Amsterdam vodka bottles.

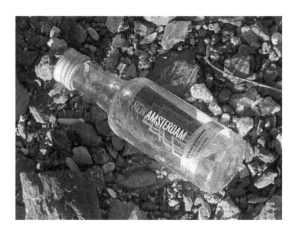

Thursday, May 28th, 2020 (Day 7 of the Arizona Walk)

Day seven's walk would take us from Camelback Ranch Glendale Stadium to Goodyear Ballpark, home of the Cincinnati Reds and Cleveland Guardians.

Vonda Vaden-Bates was back today, plus two new walkers also joined us. Carole Hemmelgarn flew in from Denver and would walk with us the last four days. Lee Perreira, known as the Marathon Man, also joined. An incredibly talented musician, Lee runs sixteen 26.2-mile runs (marathons) over sixteen straight days each year in the Arizona heat to raise money for different charities. An amazing feat!

After ten more miles of walking, we neared the front gate of Goodyear Stadium. A man in his early thirties, wearing a red polo shirt and khaki colored pants, was casually walking toward the home plate entrance gate.

Seeing our large group, he shouted, "What are you nice people doing here this morning? I hope you know the park is closed." He was not accustomed to seeing a group of people arriving at the ballpark during the pandemic.

We shared what we were doing, and he laughed. "You are all crazy!"

He told us his name was Bruce, the general manager of the ballpark.

"But I love what you were doing," he continued. "Want a quick tour of the ballpark?"

I could not get the word "absolutely" out any quicker.

Unlocking the see-through metal-wired home plate entrance gate, we followed Bruce inside and enjoyed a personalized tour of the ballpark. This was the first time I had been inside a ballpark since the pandemic started. The tiredness in my legs and body were now gone as Bruce and I talked baseball as we walked. He shared his love of the game as a child and how he found his way into baseball management. We talked for almost thirty minutes about the game we both loved, sharing stories of the Cubs–Indians 2016 World Series and his wife's secret love for the Cubs.

Driving home, I reflected about my back-and-forth baseball banter with the elderly Oakland A's fan in the parking lot at Hohokam Park, each of us sharing stories about our hometown teams. Today, it was sharing laughs and baseball stories with Bruce at Goodyear Ballpark. At this time of uncertainty and crisis across our great country, I was reminded of the Terrance Mann quote from the movie *Field of Dreams*:

"The one constant through all the years, Ray, has been baseball. America has rolled by like an army of steamrollers. It has been erased like a blackboard, rebuilt, and erased again. But baseball has marked the time. This field, this game: it is a part of our past, Ray. It reminds of us of all that once was good, and it could be again."

I hoped things could be good again.

"Time doesn't heal anything; it just teaches us
how to live with the pain."

Clearissa Lynn Castaneda

Sunday, May 31st, 2020 (Day Ten of the Arizona Walk)

Total miles walked = 597 miles
Total steps taken = 1,860,644

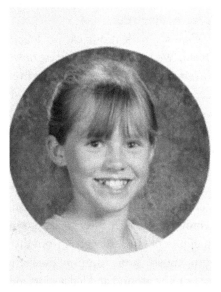

Alyssa Hemmelgarn
Photo courtesy of Carole Hemmelgarn

"Three years, seven months, and twenty-eight days"—the time it took hospital leadership to have a meaningful conversation with Carole Hemmelgarn after her daughter Alyssa died in their hospital.

Our Arizona walking days began well before sunrise to beat the heat and by now I was in a rhythm. Getting up by 3:30am had become easier if I was in bed by 8:45pm the night before and found time for a forty-five-minute afternoon nap. This morning, we were scheduled to meet an NBC news reporter at Chase Field around 5:45am. The local Arizona NBC station wanted to interview us at the start of our walk and then again when we finished at Sloan Park.

Driving back to Chase Field that morning, we had the radio on. We had just escaped getting caught up in the Black Lives Matter protests that turned to riots in downtown Phoenix the previous night and had been glued to the national news feed since George Floyd was killed in the streets of Minneapolis on May 25th, 2020. The world now was imploding and exploding, many shouting and yelling shoulder-to-shoulder at the same time we were supposed to be social distancing. We watched television reports of the rioting and looting playing out in many of the cities on my upcoming route, adding new dangers to an already foreboding year.

It was still dark when we parked our car on Jefferson Street along the north side of Chase Field. We looked east and west down Jefferson, the fluorescent streetlights illuminating an empty street. The five of us appeared to be the only people in the area, our voices echoing off the buildings. With no sign of the television news truck or the reporter who was supposed to meet us at the ballpark, we stretched our tight legs and backs near the car and lathered on sunscreen we would soon need.

Carole Hemmelgarn was walking with me again on Sunday, having flown in Wednesday evening from Denver, Colorado. Carole lost her daughter Alyssa to preventable medical harm at the age of nine and wanted to walk with me in Arizona in her memory. We walked over to the home plate entrance and gathered around a small plot of grass thirty feet from the gate. Here I pulled a bright-yellow painted memorial stone from my pocket with "Alyssa" written on it. I placed the stone on the ground and led a short memorial service in her honor. My voice began to crack in the presence of my friend Carole's grief and I had to pause between each sentence to regain my composure. I finished the memorial wiping tears from eyes, the same being true for Cathy, Vonda, and Lisa who were also walking with us today.

While hospitalized, Alyssa became seriously ill from a Clostridium dif-ficile hospital-acquired infection. Known as C. diff, approximately 200,000 cases are reported annually in U.S. hospitals. The bacterium can attack the large intestine resulting in fever, abdominal cramping, inflammation of the colon, intestinal bleeding, and dehydration. Alyssa's care team failed to rec-ognize the signs and symptoms she was experiencing or to identify critical lab results until it was too late to save her life. Similar to Lewis Blackman's catastrophic outcome, this was a classic example of "failure to rescue" that led to sepsis and contributed to her unfortunate death. In health care, it is also known as a diagnostic error or missed diagnosis. An estimated 40,000 to 80,000 patients die each year from diagnostic breakdowns in U.S. hospitals.

Carole is now a national patient safety advocate and speaker, who edu-cates hospital leaders, healthcare administrators, and health science students on how communication is key to patient-centered care and safety. Her talks help healthcare personnel become better listeners when patients and family members have concerns. She is on a personal mission to help educate others about preventable medical harm and how to stay safe when entering the healthcare system. In Carole's words, recovery from the loss of a child is never over.

Carole shared this passage about Alyssa with me:

Steps

The first step is to just get out of bed and place your feet firmly on the ground. The second is to learn to walk through life without your child. And the third is learning to run. For some it is running away from the pain, and for others, it is toward answers. For me, it took three years, seven months, and twenty-eight days of running. Running to find out what happened to my daughter.

My blonde-haired, athletic, quirky nine-year-old daughter, Alyssa, was diag-nosed with acute lymphocytic leukemia (ALL) on a Monday afternoon and died ten days later from multiple medical errors. To set the record straight, one rarely dies of ALL in ten days. Alyssa died because the culture of the organization was sick. It was a culture steeped in hierarchy, a blame-and-shame environment, and one not focused on learning.

Alyssa does not plant her feet firmly on the ground anymore, nor does she walk or run. What she leaves the world is her story. A story of recognizing diagnostic errors, implementing failure-to-rescue protocols, activating rapid response teams, and creating communication and resolution programs. She will never walk from ballpark to ballpark like Dave, or run marathons like her mom, but she is lockstep in making health care a safer place for others.

In Alyssa's medical care, the first catastrophic preventable harm was unintentional. Caregivers want to heal, not harm. However, the subsequent second harm—failing to communicate or provide answers to the Hemmelgarns for three years, seven months and twenty-eight days—was intentional, well planned, and well resourced. It is another example of the "wall of silence" hospitals and healthcare administrators build between themselves and families after medical error.

After a moment of silence, we gathered our collective resolve and began walking east. With the desert heat on its own schedule, we could not wait for the TV news team, hoping they would be waiting for us at Sloan Park. Cathy and Vonda walked with us for the first two miles before turning around and heading back to Chase Field where our car was parked. They would drive the car to mile five where we would reconnect and hydrate while grabbing a snack from our well-stocked cooler in the trunk.

When we reached mile four, my cell phone rang. It was Cathy and as soon as I answered I heard terror in her voice. She was shouting over what sounded like mayhem in the background. "It's gotten crazy back here." There were police sirens screaming in the background.

"Slow down and tell me what's going on." Unable to hear me, she continued talking over my question, her fear palpable through my phone.

"We are about two blocks from the south side of Chase Field. Storefront and restaurant windows are busted out everywhere. All the merchandise that was on display has been stolen. The sidewalk is covered with broken glass."

I was stunned. We had not seen any sign of rioting or vandalism near Chase Field when we left the downtown area.

Cathy continued talking, her words now coming in rapid fire. "There is yellow police tape over the windows. We are afraid our car may have been vandalized."

I was more worried about their safety than the car and was doing mental calculations on how long it would take us to get back to them. She was silent for at least fifteen seconds, which felt like forever with police sirens blaring through my cell phone. I asked if she was OK, but there was no answer, just more silence. Finally, she spoke.

"We made it back to the car. There are a bunch of police cars with lights flashing and a large crowd of people about four blocks down the street from where we parked. The car looks to be untouched."

Now I could hear what sounded like people chanting and screaming mixed in with the sirens.

"Get in the car and quickly drive east out of downtown. Meet us where we originally planned near mile five," I shouted through the phone.

Vonda was holding Cathy's cell phone while my wife started the car and began driving in the opposite direction of the police and protesters. I stayed on the line with them until both confirmed they were out of harm's way.

We later found out that the downtown Phoenix rioting had occurred after midnight and continued until approximately 3:30am. The NBC news crew that was supposed to meet us had been up most of the night covering the civil unrest and were catching up on much-needed sleep. We had not noticed the broken windows when we arrived because it was still dark, and we had parked on the north side of the ballpark. Most of the stores and restaurants broken into were on the south side of Chase Field. Protesters had once again assembled in the downtown area by 7:00am, at the same time Cathy and Vonda were returning to our car. The group had reassembled in the name of protest, but it felt more like an armed, angry mob than an organized, well-intended party for change. None of us were prepared to be caught up in the middle of the escalating violence.

Now that Cathy and Vonda were safe and on their way back to us, I found myself preoccupied with thoughts unrelated to patient safety for the first time since I began walking. My pace slowed, and I again fell behind Carole and Lisa. Cathy's terror and her firsthand account of the destruction and looting had me unsettled in ways I could not place. The peaceful protests Saturday evening had turned ugly in the early morning hours with hoodlum looters destroying businesses, public buildings, and the ballpark. To me, the term "peaceful protest" has become an oxymoron, especially when race or religion is the focus of the protest. The intent of some protesters involved may be peaceful but political polarization and social media misinformation attracts opportunists looking for confrontation, arriving at a peaceful protest in full protective gear and holding AK-47s.

Images of the gray Dodge Challenger accelerating into a crowd of protesters in Charlottesville, Virginia on Saturday, August 12th, 2017, killing one woman and injuring over thirty others, replaced thoughts about where our next rest stop would be. The "Unite the Right" protest and march organized by neo-Nazis, white supremacists, and Ku Klux Klan members in response to the removal of a Robert E. Lee statue was never meant to be peaceful; the intent was to incite and confront. Blog posts leading up to the rally called for confrontation and asked people to come armed and ready to fight. Many of the protesters arriving in the park were wearing combat gear, holding white nationalist banners and Nazi flags with swastikas on them, chanting "blood and soil," a World War II Nazi slogan intended to highlight the racial purity of German people and their connection to the German homeland. Civil rights counter-protesters who heard about their intentions also showed up in Charlottesville armed and ready for confrontation. Lines in the sand were drawn and when the white supremacists attempted to march, they were confronted by the counter-protesters. Violent fights broke out in the streets between the two factions.

A block behind the others now, my mind continued to drift back to 1977, when my hometown of Skokie became known for something its Jewish residents had most feared. The American neo-Nazis chose Skokie as the site for a march because there were still many Holocaust survivors living there, proving that antisemitism, like racism, was still alive and well. The exact reason my family and my friends' families had settled in the quiet suburb now put a bullseye on the forehead of every Jew living peacefully in our growing community. The neo-Nazis wanted to intimidate and threaten Jews around the world by marching through our streets dressed in the same German military uniforms adorned with swastikas and worn by the Nazi soldiers during World War II. Six million Jewish people were slaughtered through religious genocide by Hitler and the Nazi regime during World War II, and these people wanted to celebrate this massacre on the same streets we worked, prayed, and played on each day. Parents, siblings, cousins, and friends of those now living in Skokie had been violently murdered during the Holocaust. By marching in Skokie, the neo-Nazis were forcing our family, friends, and neighbors to relive the horrors so many in our community refused to speak of, let alone put out for public display.

After lengthy court battles, the march was moved to Chicago and pushed to April 1978, though the emotional damage to those living in Skokie had been done. News outlets across the country reported on the march, which only aided the neo-Nazis in achieving their goal of inflicting pain on Holocaust survivors and Jews in Skokie and around the world. In 1981, this story was retold with the release of the movie *Skokie*, written by Ernest Kinoy and directed by Herbert Wise, which included a star-studded, classic cast of Danny Kaye, Carl Reiner, Eli Wallach, and Brian Dennehy. The overarching message of Kinoy's script is that Jews who turned the other cheek instead of standing up to fight made Hitler's intentions easier to realize. The intimidation and persecution had to stop. I had come to believe, especially considering the televised events since George Floyd's murder, that there is never a peaceful protest when religious bigotry or racial injustice are involved; the confrontation always turns ugly.

I took deep breaths to slow my racing heart and sipped on my water bottle, trying to check my emotions before picking up my pace to catch up with our group, who was waiting for me at a busy intersection. We continued our own peaceful march for patient safety, now passing a strip club on East Washington Street at about mile six which provided some much-needed levity. The ladies had fun camping in front of the large neon sign and we captured some fun moments of our team in action, in contrast to the photos Cathy and Vonda had taken of the destruction less than an hour earlier.

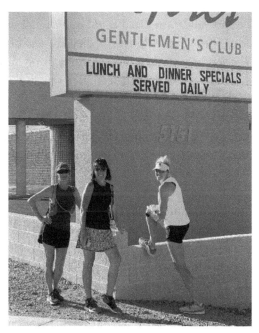

Barbara, Lisa and Carole
Photo courtesy of Dave Mayer (2020)

By mile eight, we were back in Tempe, walking on newly paved sidewalks in a college town where all of us felt less threatened. Rioters and broken glass were miles behind us, at least for now, despite the world still spinning on a tilt. The comfort of friendship and our shared mission provided protection from all the uncertainty being projected from our phones and televisions. Our last three miles were more lighthearted and less taxing, our route taking us through the Arizona State University (ASU) campus along a reservoir where we watched rowing teams going through their morning workouts, and then on past the ASU football stadium, the west-side grandstands built into the side of a small mountain.

About 1.5 miles from Sloan Park, we could see the light towers of the ballpark in the distance. It was now time to unfold our ten-foot by three-foot Patient Safety Movement Foundation banner. Everyone held a portion of the long sign that forced us from the sidewalk and onto Rio Salado Parkway, growing closer to the finish line. The NBC TV reporter showed up, apologizing for the team's absence this morning, and then walked the final mile with us while filming and asking questions along the way.

I felt my heart racing when we reached Sloan Park, not from dehydration but from gratitude and validation that I could pull this all off. If I could survive ten days walking through the Phoenix Valley, the rest of my route would be much easier. The reporter stuck his microphone in my face, the spotlight now on me, and asked, "How do you feel after walking 125 miles in the desert sun?"

The only words I could find were, "I'm tired!" Forrest Gump immediately came to mind, this being the same explanation his character gave when he stopped running. I was momentarily speechless, taking in all we had just accomplished and been through.

Our Phoenix walk had turned out to be 135 miles, which was ten miles longer than our original route. Though not a healthcare professional or patient advocate in the formal sense, our friend Lisa Riegle had walked all ten days, never once complaining about the heat, my miscalculated mileage, the road conditions, or the threats to personal safety. My wife, Cathy, not only walked most of the 135 miles, but she also served as our sag wagon director, cook, and coach. Barbara, Carole, Vonda, and Lee, who joined me on days they were in Phoenix, made up our small but mighty team of passionate and committed people trying to make a difference.

Walking around Sloan Park one last time before heading home, I visited the memorial stone we had left for Michael Skolnik ten days earlier. I was encouraged to see that the stone was still lying in the grass garden by the home plate gate where we had left it. We were making a mark after all.

The NBC sportscaster who interviewed us that afternoon had taken our mission to heart. The piece he cut together on my walk captured the urgency of our patient safety mission, as well as Carole's and Vonda's personal stories, and the depth of what we had just accomplished. The media coverage in Phoenix had been more than I had expected with all four local TV stations airing two-minute morning and evening news segments on my walk, two live radio interviews, and a featured *Arizona Republic* newspaper article. My walk in the Phoenix Valley only reinforced my passion, and I was now ready to take my walk across America on the road to further raise awareness of the need to improve healthcare safety.

"No Safety, Know Pain. Know Safety, No Pain."

Author unknown

Wednesday, June 24th, 2020

Total Miles Walked = 874
Total Steps = 2,223,614

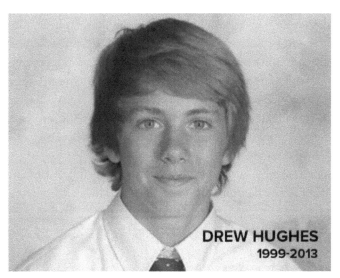

Drew Hughes
Photo courtesy of the Patient Safety Movement Foundation

Drew Hughes could light up a room with his charisma and good looks. He was a heartwarming young man who loved grabbing his mitt and heading to Western

Park looking for a baseball game. Drew was very athletic, playing Pop-Warner Football for the Newport Vikings, as well as football and basketball at Broad Creek Middle School, where he also starred as a member of the track team.

Drew Hughes died at the age of thirteen from preventable medical harm. He suffered a concussion from a skateboard accident and was electively intubated as a precautionary measure for transport to a second hospital. He was not sedated properly, waking up during the transport confused and pulling his breathing tube out. A paramedic on the ambulance gave Drew a paralytic agent before reintubating him. When they reinserted his breathing tube, they incorrectly placed the tube in his esophagus, not his trachea. Drew went for thirty minutes without oxygen before they realized their mistake, which resulted in his tragic death.

A thirteen-year-old child should never die from preventable medical harm. Unlike me, who dreamed of playing center field for the Chicago Cubs but lacked athletic talent, Drew had that talent and might have played professional baseball. However, Drew's parents were deprived of seeing that dream come true for their son.

Two days from today, I would be walking in Denver in memory of Drew Hughes. It would be the seventh anniversary of his death, and I was thinking about Drew and his love of baseball as we pulled out of our garage at 4:30am on June 24th. We were ready to begin our cross-country road trip to visit the remaining twenty-eight Major League ballparks while walking with family and friends who had lost loved ones to medical error in those same cities. The trip would span almost three months, and our route would put 15,000 miles on our little Audi coupe turned tiny camper.

My high beams lit up the road and caught a large, black animal scurrying in front of the car. I slammed on my brakes, sending Cathy flying into her seatbelt, which thankfully kept her from hitting the dashboard. Her piercing scream broke the silence of the early morning hour, and I fully expected to see nearby house lights flipped on.

"What on Earth are you doing?" she yelled.

"I almost hit a field rat the size of a cat!" This was not a good omen for the start of our trip.

"Next time, just hit it! Those rats get into garbage cans," she said. "And don't even start thinking it is bad luck! I know you."

"It's good luck because I missed it. That thing was huge!"

My wife knew me. Like baseball players and professional athletes, anesthesiologists and surgeons are often tied to talismans that ensure success. Whether a lucky scrub cap, a particular song played just before the first incision is made, or an anesthesia cart arranged just so—we all had a need for ritual and routine in common.

Being a Cubs fan, I have a right to be superstitious. True diehards have endured the Billy Goat Curse, coming back year after year to Wrigley Field, known as the World's Biggest Outdoor Beer Garden, to root for our hometown heroes—win or lose. The curse had been placed on the Cubs in 1945 by William Sianis, a Greek immigrant who had purchased the Lincoln Tavern on West Madison Avenue across the street from the Chicago Stadium in 1934 for $205. Sianis later renamed it the Billy Goat Tavern after he adopted a kid billy goat that had been left on the doorstep of the establishment. When the Cubs played the Detroit Tigers in the 1945 World Series, a season when the only playoff games were the World Series, sports fan and marketer Sianis bought two box-seat tickets and attended the game held at Wrigley Field with his pet billy goat. While competing versions of the story exist, both narratives agree that Sianis and his goat were asked to leave—either because the goat was bothering fans, or because P.K. Wrigley said the goat smelled. Enraged, Sianis allegedly declared, "Them Cubs! They ain't gonna win no more!" His words turned to truth when the Cubs lost the 1945 World Series, and the losing streak continued.

Cathy and I settled back into our seats, both of us silent as I merged onto Highway 303. I prayed that would be the last animal of any size to dart into our path. My thoughts took me to Shea Stadium, 1969, when the Cubs played the Mets. On August 19th, with six weeks left in the regular season, the Cubs led the National League division by eight games, with the Mets a safe distance behind in second place. By September 9th, their lead dwindled to 1.5 games, after losing the first game of the series to the Mets 3–2 on a disputed call at home plate. In the top of the first inning of the second game, with Billy Williams at bat and Ron Santo in the on-deck circle, a New York fan trying to rattle the team released a black cat in front of the Cubs dugout.

A Cubs' batboy at the time, Jim Flood, was interviewed by *Sports Illustrated* about the event and recalled watching the cat creep toward Cubs manager Leo Durocher seated in the dugout. "He was saying, 'Somebody get that cat outta here. Get him away from me!' I didn't know if I should laugh or what. I mean, I was a kid. But we were playing like crap, and now this. I do not know if it was because of the cat but we played terrible after that. The Mets blew right past us."[6]

The rest is in the history books. That year, the Cubs lost seventeen of their last twenty-five games, helping the "Miracle Mets," who won twenty-three of their last thirty games, clinch the division title on September 24th, while earning the well-known moniker by baseball fans.

I missed sitting in the bleachers, enjoying a Vienna hot dog on a poppy seed bun and watching a baseball game. With the season on hold, it felt reassuring to go back in time and relive America's national pastime. On Monday, June 24th, there was a glimmer of hope for the 2020 season when baseball players agreed to a shortened, sixty-game schedule for 2020. Baseball would officially start on July 23rd after a few weeks of summer camp, in place of spring training so that players could get their bodies in baseball condition. All games would be played in empty stadiums to keep players healthy and the public safe.

After seven hours of driving, we arrived for an overnight stay in Santa Fe, New Mexico, located in the foothills of the Sangre de Cristo Mountains. After checking into our hotel, we headed out for a five-mile walk through the city. A lover of southwest culture, I slowed my pace to admire the Pueblo-styled light-brown clay and stone single-story buildings and southwest art galleries lining the streets adjacent to Santa Fe Plaza. An early evening margarita in a decoratively painted sixteen-ounce glass followed by a sizzling platter of steak fajitas at an outdoor café completed a perfect first day of travel. It was the first time Cathy and I had eaten at a restaurant since the pandemic started. Tomorrow, we would complete our drive to Denver, Colorado, staying with our daughter Tracy and her family.

After another seven hours of driving, we arrived at our daughter's home in Highlands Ranch, a suburb of Denver. Our plan included a two-day walk from Red Rocks Park located in the foothills of the Rocky Mountains, ending the next day at Coors Field located in downtown Denver. That gave us a little less than twenty-four hours to acclimate to the Mile High City before heading above 6,450 feet. I've lived my entire life at sea level, from Chicago to

---

[6] Lucas, Paul. 'It's My One Claim to Fame": The Untold Story of the Cubs Black Cat Jinx. www.si.com. September 6th, 2019.

Baltimore to Phoenix. My first few hours in Colorado always left me gasping for breath.

Early Friday morning, June 29th, Cathy, Tracy, and I met up with Carole Hemmelgarn, who lives in Denver. Carole had walked with me the last four days in Phoenix and was joining us again to memorialize her daughter, Alyssa, who died from preventable medical harm at the age of nine. At the main entrance to Red Rocks National Park, we also met up with Dr. Arthur "Art" Kanowitz, an emergency room physician and founder of the Airway Safety Movement. Art was walking in memory of Drew Hughes, the thirteen-year-old boy who lost his life to preventable medical harm, who was also the son of his good friend, David Hughes.

Before starting down the trail that morning, I stopped to admire the beauty of our surroundings. The entire 738-acre park filled with hiking trails and wildlife is located on the eastern slope of the Rocky Mountains just fifteen miles west of downtown Denver. The Red Rocks Amphitheater, which opened in 1941, is easily considered to be one of the best venues in the world to see a concert, especially during the summer months. Watching the setting sun bounce off the red sandstone while it mixes with the band's light show in this intimate setting is something every music fan needs to experience.

We had the park to ourselves, despite the need to start hikes early in Colorado so as not to get caught in summer thunderstorms and, more importantly, to avoid the afternoon lightning. Stopping halfway up one of the well-worn gravel trails, I admired the panoramic view the elevation afforded us in the area named a National Historic Landmark in 2015. As we continued zig-zagging across the red, orange, and brown silt-covered paths running between boulders the size of small trucks, I began to see the outline of downtown Denver. The city's modern, manufactured steel and glass high-rise buildings were dwarfed by the rock formations, known as the ancestral Rockies, which surrounded me. With downtown Denver, the flat great plains, and the rising morning sun off to the east and a row of 14,000-foot snow-capped Rocky Mountain peaks off to the west, this was truly nature at its best. I breathed in the fresh mountain air, the smell of sagebrush and wildflowers tickling my nose. Energized by nature's majestic powers, I was now ready to lead the group on to Coors Field, and even happier to be descending versus ascending the 1,200 feet down to the Mile High City.

Two renowned patient safety educators, Shelly Dierking and Dr. Wendy Madigosky, a family medicine physician, joined our Colorado group. The sky was a perfect Cubby blue. The scattered morning clouds disappeared, leaving the heat of the morning sun. A grey hawk circled our group overhead, floating upon currents of air while hunting for its first prey of the day. Tall pine trees lined our trail, also serving as a shady sanctuary for small herds of deer feeding on tall grass. After two hours of walking, we came across a creek that now ran alongside our trail, none of us able to resist dipping our hands into the ice-cold water flowing from the snow-capped mountains behind us. The peaceful, rhythmic sound of the rushing water pulled us all into silent reflection as we made our way to the day's twelve-mile finish line. A local FOX TV reporter was waiting to interview us at the entrance to the small park where we finished, spending time talking with Carole about her daughter Alyssa. The segment featuring Carole appeared on the local evening news that night.

Once the interview had finished, we made our way to a quiet area in the park to hold a short moment of silence for Drew Hughes.

David Hughes shared the following passage with me about his son Drew:

It seems cliché, but Drew was one of those kids who lit up a room when he walked in. It is so sad that in so many cases of children leaving us too soon that seems to be a pervasive sentiment. In our family, he was the puzzle piece that completed the picture. Drew managed to fill a needed spot in our family. He made me, my wife, and his brother better people, and what he added to all our lives is even more noticeable now that he's gone. Drew was completely comfortable in his skin and what others thought never really mattered. I think that characteristic above many was one of the reasons he was so well-liked by his peers and everyone he met. Even in the briefest encounters he made a lasting impression on those he spoke to. In all aspects of his life, it seemed his main purpose was to make other people happy. It is exceedingly difficult to encapsulate Drew in a paragraph, and I could write so much more, but I believe this is enough. As his father, and after the many stories we have heard from others over the years, I genuinely believe Drew accomplished in a short nearly fourteen years what many hope to achieve in a full lifetime.

On June 28th, 2013, Drew suffered a head injury and mild concussion while skateboarding with his friends. I worked at the local hospital and told my wife to just bring him there, and I would meet them in the ED. I walked to the ED and told the staff that my son was being brought in and that I wanted him transferred to a different hospital that had a higher level of care, should it be needed. After Drew arrived, a CT scan was performed. The results were normal, but they suspected a basilar skull fracture. I was by Drew's side the entire time he was in the ED and we spoke about what was going on and that I knew he was OK. He was scared, but he was calm and reassured with me by his side. After some time of working out the logistics, the decision was made to transport Drew via the hospital's EMS service. I would be unable to ride in the ambulance with him and the ED physician told me she wanted to sedate and intubate Drew for the hour-and-a-half trip as a precautionary measure. He was anxious when me or my wife were not with him, and she felt it would be best. Drew would sleep for the trip and we would follow the ambulance in our personal vehicle. There are many details to what happened with Drew, but I will get to the events that ended his life. Drew was not sedated properly for a child his age and very shortly after beginning the transport Drew woke up and began pulling out his ET tube. The paramedic on the ambulance with Drew administered vecuronium (a paralytic) to control Drew and no further sedation was administered. They bagged Drew for five minutes in which he was awake and paralyzed before reintubating him. When they reintubated Drew they placed the tube in his esophagus, and he began suffocating immediately. Drew went for nearly thirty minutes without oxygen before they stopped at a closer hospital en route and the esophageal intubation was recognized. The tube placement was corrected, but at this point he had severe hypoxic brain damage and when he arrived at the hospital where we were waiting, he had no brain activity. We stopped life support and Drew passed away the following day, June 29th, 2013.

Have you ever watched a movie where a child died? Or saw it on the news—with a clip of the devastated mother or other family members? Or even had a friend or an acquaintance that lost a child? And you let your brain go to that place where you thought how you would react or feel if that were you and your child was suddenly gone? And you thought, "Oh my gosh, I would not survive it, I'd curl up in a ball and stay there forever ... they'd have to put me in a mental hospital. . . ." But then you just had to shift your brain to something else because it was far too much to bear or to even think about, so you said a quick prayer for this other family and also a prayer of thanksgiving for your healthy, living children. Secretly, you were so glad it was them and not you. I mean God doesn't give us more than we can bear, right? And you know you couldn't bear that so you had a false confidence that it would never happen to you. We were those people and yes, it hurts just as bad as you imagined it would. We would not have ever thought we were strong enough to continue living without one of our children, but we are surviving. With Drew's two older brothers, their families, and now grandchildren, we are moving forward, but there is always that missing puzzle piece. The hardest part is knowing *that if one thing had been done correctly in the back of that ambulance that puzzle piece would still be in its place, where it's supposed to be....*

Airway management is something anesthesiologists do very adeptly every day. When others must do the same, with less frequency or experience, it can get tricky. Safely managing and monitoring a patient's airway when they are unable to manage their own airway during surgery or because of illness or injury is a critical skill. Airway safety events can occur during the active management of a patient's airway when the intubation fails or is delayed, when the intubation tube is poorly placed—as in Drew's case—or when pressure injuries, aspiration, and unplanned extubations occur. These safety events can lead to complications such as hypoxemia, vocal cord injury, tissue ulceration, pneumonia, brain injury and in the worst case, death. Some estimates put the annual death rate from airway management errors at over 30,000 patients. Using evidenced-based, best-practice guidelines and protocols, and calling for assistance when needed, preventable airway management deaths can be reduced to zero. What happened to Drew should never have happened, and our walk in Colorado honored his young life.

"Don't harm me, heal me, treat me well."

Original author unknown

Day two in Colorado began where we had finished the previous day, twelve miles from our destination of Coors Field. Today, Deahna Visscher also joined our walking team. Deahna had lost her son Grant when he was eleven days old because of preventable medical harm. We would remember Grant at Coors Field with a memorial rock ceremony later in the day.

A highlight of our second day in Colorado was that our son-in-law Josh and our two granddaughters, Ellie and Lainey, joined us to walk the last four miles to Coors Field. Continuing along the dirt trail that ran alongside the South Platte River into downtown Denver, the quietness of the foothills was replaced by the sounds of trucks and cars speeding into the city on Interstate 25 fifty yards to the right of us. An NBC TV news reporter filmed our group as we approached Coors Field. Carole, Art, and Deahna led the way, holding our PSMF banner the last half mile before finishing at Coors Field. The team celebrated completion of our twenty-four-mile walk in front of a bronze statue entitled "The Player," created by sculptor George Lundeen, which stands in front of the main gate to Coors Field. The statue is a tribute to Hall of Famer Wesley "Branch" Rickey, who had a short-lived playing career from 1905 to '07 and is best known for his accomplishments as a baseball executive. It was Rickey who launched the farm system for up-and-coming ballplayers, and who strongly opposed baseball's color barrier. He was also an innovator and leader who signed Jackie Robinson to a minor league contract in 1945, and who later shepherded Robinson, the first Black player to play Major League Baseball, to his debut with the Brooklyn Dodgers in 1947.

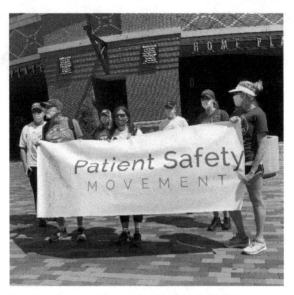

Art, Deahna, and Carole holding the PSMF banner
Photo courtesy of Dave Mayer (2020)

Deahna, Carole, and Art were interviewed by the reporter, sharing why each walked with me. They shared personal insights about Grant, Alyssa, and Drew and how the healthcare system failed to protect them. The reporter also filmed the memorial rock service and moment of silence we had for Alyssa, Grant, and Drew. Here, we again placed three painted memorial stones, each with one of the children's names written upon it, in the garden just west of the main gate. Watching the segment on Denver's ten o'clock news that night, the three different stories of preventable loss helped educate the public about medical errors.

Deahna shared this passage with me about her son Grant:

Grant was our surprise baby. Surprised we got pregnant so quickly with him. Surprised that he was going to be born with a heart defect. Surprised that he arrived three weeks early. Surprised that he would be going home just over a week after having open heart surgery. Surprised that he died from a preventable medical error when he was only eleven days old.

We went into Grant's pregnancy with hope and fear of the unknown. We went through it with wonder and amazement at the advancement of science and medicine. We came out of it with devastation and despair.

I had difficulty getting pregnant with our first child, so it was unexpected that we became pregnant with our second child. At eighteen weeks gestation, we learned our son would be born with a heart defect. Grant arrived on April 8th, 2008, with coarctation of the aorta. He had open heart surgery on April 12th, 2008. The following week doctors and nurses were impressed with how quickly he was recovering and told us that we would be going home soon. This is why it was such a shock that on the night of April 19th, 2008, he died before our eyes while over twenty medical professions tried to resuscitate him.

Earlier that day a nurse was not comfortable with Grant's feeding tube, so she put in a new one. When she struggled to insert the new feeding tube, I asked her questions about her verification technique. I had no idea that the questions I was asking then would foreshadow the events that followed. All day long we watched Grant struggle. He blew milky white bubbles that throughout the day the nurses had to suction out. His monitors kept alarming. Worse was his coloring, his skin starting to look pale and grey. That night, a code blue was called to his room.

We never knew such despair until that night. My husband and I collapsed to the floor in deep, gut-wrenching sobs when the doctors told us that Grant had died. Later that night we learned he died because the nurse misplaced his feeding tube. In the weeks that followed we learned that was a very preventable medical error. We were both shocked, hurt, and angered. Those emotions later turned into a driving force and need to change our outcome for others. It was then that I decided that no one else should suffer the loss of a child or family member due to a preventable medical error. That is why today I continue to fight for patient safety. The road is long, there is still a lot of work to do, but I know that someday we will reach zero harm.

Misplaced nasogastric and other types of feeding tubes pose a serious threat to patient safety because the error can cause serious harm or death. While no method for assuring proper placement of a feeding tube is 100 percent foolproof, the *Patient Safety Advisor*, produced by the Pennsylvania Patient Safety Authority in collaboration with the ECRI Institute and Institute for Safe Medication Practices, recommends several strategies that can help reduce harm. A few of these recommendations include: 1) using a feeding tube only when medically indicated; 2) using radiographic confirmation of tube placement when available; 3) developing policies and procedures that enforce standardization of best practices; and 4) ensuring that healthcare providers have proven competencies in tube placement and verification of location.

Family members should also play an active role on the feeding tube team. In Grant's situation, Deahna and her husband were at their son's bedside, sensed something was wrong, and shared their concerns with members of Grant's care team. Unfortunately, their concerns were not acknowledged.

After an emotional two days in Denver, Cathy and I were back on the road Sunday morning, July 1st, on our way to Kansas City for a six-mile walk to Kauffman Stadium, home of the Kansas City Royals that would also include a walk around Arrowhead Stadium, home of the Kansas City Chiefs football team. A true sports fan, I could not pass up the chance to see both historic stadiums while in town. The next day, we headed to St. Louis for another long walk to Busch Stadium, home of the Cubs' longtime rival, the St. Louis Cardinals.

In front of Busch Stadium stood a full roster of eight-foot-tall bronze action statues paying homage to Cardinal legends and Hall of Famers. Stan "The Man" Musial, Enos Slaughter, Dizzy Dean, Rogers Hornsby, Red Schoendienst, Lou Brock, Bob Gibson, and Ozzie Smith, to name a few. The statues brought back memories of growing up a Cubs fan. Pitching duels between Bob Gibson, the Cardinals star pitcher who won 251 games, a two-time winner of the Cy Young Award, and Fergie Jenkins, the Cubs pitching ace who won twenty games over six consecutive seasons and claimed the Cy Young Award in 1971. Today, starting pitchers go five to six innings and then head to the showers. Gibson and Jenkins refused to give up the baseball, pitching ten innings or more on many occasions.

Cubs fans never forget the one-sided trade that sent future Hall of Famer Lou Brock to the Cardinals for Ernie Broglio (yes, you can say it: who?) and listening to games called by legendary broadcasters Jack Buck, Jack Brickhouse, and Harry Caray, three of the best in the business. Jack Buck's "That's a winner!" closing after each Cardinals victory. Jack Brickhouse's "Hey, Hey" after each Cubs' home run, the most memorable being his call of Ernie Banks 500th homer into the left field bleachers at Wrigley Field. And what baseball fan didn't sing along with Harry Caray's "Take me out to the ballgame" during the seventh inning stretch? The rivalry between the St. Louis Cardinals and Chicago Cubs remains one of the best in sports.

About an hour east of St. Louis on I-70, I was humming along to Jimmy Buffett singing "One Particular Harbor" on Margaritaville Radio. Cathy was dozing beside me, so I had control of the radio once again. If it were up to me,

I would have had Jimmy Buffet serenade us across the country, but my wife liked to switch it up. She stirred in her seat, opened her eyes, and pointed at the gas gauge.

"We need to stop and fill up. You know I hate it when you run the gas tank down to less than a quarter of a tank." That she could shift from sleep to wakefulness and be so aware of her surroundings was a result of having been a nurse for over thirty years.

This was at least the third time since leaving Denver that she had urged me to fill up. I liked to wait until the needle hit "empty" on the gauge, confident I still had about two gallons left to find the next gas station. Unlike health care, auto makers understand human factors and design accordingly. They know people like me push the limit and on a rare occasion will run out of gas, so they design a gas tank to register empty when there are still a couple of gallons left in the tank. From my viewpoint, I try to optimize the number of miles per tank of gas in order to reduce the number of stops we had to make; the less contact with others during the pandemic, the better.

"It's all farmland here. It could be forty miles before the next gas station!"

The gas gauge showed less than an eighth of a tank left. "We have plenty of gas," I said, then wondered how many times we had this same conversation over our thirty-two years of marriage.

Not wanting to push our luck or irritate Cathy, I exited I-70 at the Vandalia, Illinois, exit and felt her relax next to me. I pulled into the first minimart gas station and, after fueling the tank, I decided to use the bathroom and restock our cooler. Approaching the entrance, I was comforted to see the two, now ubiquitous, large signs on the sliding glass door. The first read "Face Masks Required" and the second was a graphic with two stick-figure people standing arms-length apart to encourage social distancing. It was reassuring that most gas stations and restaurants were adhering to the mask mandate issued by the CDC to keep customers safe, so that they could remain open.

Once inside the minimart, however, I couldn't help but notice I was the only one wearing a mask. About a dozen people, the largest crowd I had seen gathered in months, stood shoulder-to-shoulder without masks at the deli counter, waiting to order sandwiches. As I passed the large group, several customers glared at me, making me uncomfortable that a confrontation was imminent. I avoided further eye contact, looking at the menu sign posted behind the counter, before turning around and exiting the minimart.

This was the first time since leaving Arizona that I sensed my mask was a trigger to those around me. I may as well have been waving a matador's bright red cape; it felt like I was provoking something negative by following good public health policy. It was also the first time in almost 1,000 miles of driving that I feared for my safety because I chose to wear a mask.

It was becoming evident that the political divide in the United States was only widening, with those on either extreme becoming more entrenched in their beliefs, especially when it came to how the virus was being managed. Driving through America's heartland, we were beginning to witness the differences in those beliefs.

"It's 106 miles to Chicago, we've got a full tank, half pack of cigarettes, it's dark out, and we're wearing sunglasses. Hit it."

Jake and Elwood Blues, The Blues Brothers

Wednesday, July 2nd, 2020

Total Miles Walked = 928
Total Steps = 2,350,255

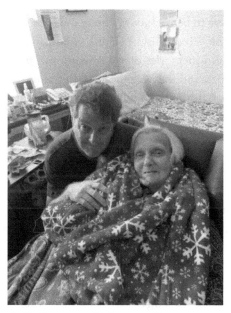

Judie Burrows with her son Steve
Photo courtesy of Steve Burrows

In 2009, at the age of sixty-nine years, Judie Burrows was admitted to a Milwaukee hospital after fracturing her hip while riding her bike. She waited eight days in the hospital in excruciating pain with no plan of care before finally being rushed into the operating room for surgery. Judie had been taking a drug called clopidogrel, a blood thinner also known as Plavix. Guidelines from the American College of Surgeons at the time recommended stopping Plavix five to seven days before surgery to reduce the risk of excessive bleeding. In Judie's case, the hospital continued giving her the blood-thinning drug over her eight-day stay in the hospital, as well as two other blood thinners. During a two-hour hip surgery that would eventually last six hours, Judie lost more than half of her five-liter blood volume, requiring multiple transfusions. She left the operating room in a coma and was taken to an e-intensive care unit (EICU) where she lay, her blood pressure, heart rate, and other critical vital signs presumably being monitored by a physician sitting in an office near the Milwaukee airport, miles from the hospital.

Over the last few years, I have become good friends with Steve and Margo Burrows and was excited to be spending time with them in two days.

We arrived in the Chicago suburbs in the late afternoon on Wednesday, July 2nd. It was great to be back in my hometown, having spent almost sixty years of my life in the Windy City. As Frank Sinatra said, Chicago is "my kind of town." I have fond memories of the museums, restaurants, sports teams, lakefront and beaches, and the Magnificent Mile, and was excited to be walking this coming week through the suburbs I grew up in before finishing at the "Friendly Confines" of Wrigley Field.

True to summer in Chicago, temperatures were in the high eighties and the air thick with humidity when we pulled into the empty Fairfield Inn parking lot in Deerfield, Illinois, our home for the next ten days. The weed-infested, yellow, burned-out grass surrounding the hotel was knee high and had not been cut in at least a month, and only one car was parked at the back of the expansive black asphalt parking lot. The hotel looked shut down—more like Alfred Hitchcock's Bates Motel than a steadfast Marriott property whose amenities were consistently good, a chain we had come to depend on when on the road.

I was relieved to see two large "Face Masks Required" signs posted on the sliding glass door at the entrance of the hotel. The words were printed in black below the word "HEALTH." Two additional red-and-white signs indicated the social distancing requirements inside the property. The images depicted a man and woman drawn in black with an arrow on both sides and the number 6 in the center. This relieved me to an extent, but I remined skeptical given the contradictions of signage and behavior that had played out in southern Illinois.

The overhead lights had been turned off in the lobby. Dispensers with handwipes sticking out the top were mounted on both sides of the entrance door. Sunlight peeked through the glass doors behind me and we saw no sign of travelers, housekeepers, or valets to assist with our luggage. A young woman wearing a face mask emerged from the office and took her place behind the erected eight-foot-tall plexiglass screen that wrapped around the check-in counter. Additional warning signs about face masks and social distancing were posted on both sides of the wall. I stood, as directed, on an orange plastic circle glued to the floor six feet from the counter, knowing we were the only people in this hotel lobby.

The hotel employee restarted her idle computer and said "Welcome to the Fairfield Inn. Are you checking in?" Between her mask, our separation, and the barrier, a two-way conversation became a guessing game.

"I am," I replied with a smile, raising my driver's license next to my face as proof of my identity—forgetting for a moment that most of my face was hidden. I hoped she could read the small font from where she was standing. We were beginning to see the way of the COVID-19-induced impersonal world, and since few people were traveling, we were inadvertently helping Marriott work out the kinks.

She located my reservation and instructed me to slide my credit card into the chip reader affixed to a small metal table next to the check-in counter. After finishing the check-in process on the computer, she grabbed her phone and looked up.

"Your room key will be accessible through the hotel app on your phone," she said, pointing at her phone to guide me. "You pretty much have the place to yourselves. Only two other parties are staying with us."

The empty parking lot suggested that we might be one of few staying on the property, but her admission caught me by surprise. This meant that with 140 hotel rooms, only three were occupied. I wanted to ask her what normal occupancy at this time of year should be, Deerfield being less than thirty miles from downtown Chicago and near several corporate headquarters of biotech and manufacturing companies but decided against trying to struggle through that conversation.

Walking back to the car to collect our bags, I contemplated the polar opposite adherence to COVID-19 precautions we observed between Vandalia and Deerfield, both cities in the same state with the same governor and just a short four-hour drive separating the two towns. That people were making up their rules in the middle of a pandemic was not surprising.

We'd been wearing masks for most of our trip and couldn't wait to get in the room and discard them. We'd Lysol-wipe all touch areas in the bedroom, bathroom, closet, and drawer space before unpacking and relaxing. This was a ritual Cathy and I followed—a type of protocol at each hotel we stayed at during our trip. We'd step into the room, set down our luggage, and begin disinfecting countertops, nightstands, TVs, and door knobs.

Cathy and I were thrilled to be within striking distance of our son Scott and his family. It had been eight months since we had seen him, his wife Leah, and our two grandchildren, Brody and Joelle. Like many, the pandemic had made family time a virtual get-together. We were also happy to be off the road and stretched out for a good night's sleep and a day with our family before driving to Milwaukee's American Family Fields ballpark. The meteorologist on the ten o'clock news predicted an excessive heat warning for the week ahead with temperatures in the mid-nineties, with intermittent thunderstorms peppering the seven-day forecast and adding to the challenge of our one-hundred-mile walk from Milwaukee to Wrigley Field.

Sunday, July 5th, 2020 (Day One)

After a bitter cup of coffee brewed in the hotel room coffee maker, we were on the road driving north to Milwaukee's American Family Fields, arriving at the ballpark just before 7:00am, where Steve and Margo Burrows were waiting for us. Steve's distinguished long, curly hair was visible under his Green Bay Packers baseball cap. Margo was leaning on two crutches and sporting an above-the-ankle boot cast, having recently broken a bone in her foot. Steve and Margo had written, directed, and produced the HBO award-winning, critically acclaimed documentary *Bleed Out*, which chronicles the ten-year battle and eventual death of Steve's mother, Judie, after preventable medical harm.

"Welcome to Milwaukee!" Steve yelled, giving me a big fist pump in the air as soon as I stepped out of the car. Steve and Margo had been splitting their time between their Hollywood home and Milwaukee, living in the home Steve grew up in while taking care of his mother before she passed away.

I was fortunate to have met Judie Burrows at the Milwaukee Film Fest when *Bleed Out* was shown to a standing-room-only audience in October 2019, three months before her death. Sitting in a wheelchair and wrapped in a thick red blanket at the back of the theater, the years of pain and suffering had taken their toll on this once beautiful woman who was vibrant and active before her tragic surgery. Despite her frail appearance, she smiled at all the well-wishers who stopped and said hello.

Steve shared the following passage about his mother Judie:

In 2009, my mom, Judie Burrows, a retired special education schoolteacher, went in for a routine partial hip replacement and came out in a coma with permanent brain damage. My uncle, a doctor, and my aunt, a nurse, told me to get the medical records ASAP. Within minutes of reviewing the surgical records, my doctor uncle discovered my mom had lost over one-half the blood in her body during this botched surgery. He also uncovered that the anesthesia records had been falsified. He ordered me to become power of attorney, to get the medical records before the hospital changed them again and to get an attorney, that this was not only medical malpractice but an intentional cover-up.

And thus began my family's decade-long journey into medical, legal, and financial hell.

My mom's cognitive and physical injuries due to loss of oxygen to the brain were profound, severe, and irreversible. She would experience incalculable pain and suffering for the next ten years, eventually succumbing in 2020 to the injuries inflicted upon her. At no time was the hospital and/or the doctors accountable or transparent. No apologies were ever given. Our only recourse to get the truth about what had happened was to go to court, which would take seven years and a quarter of $1 million.

Other than my mom's horrific suffering, seeing doctors lie under oath at trial was the single worst thing I have ever experienced in my life. I had also discovered this hospital system had replaced bedside intensive care doctors with cameras that weren't on. Then I discovered that medical error is the third leading cause of death in America. This was simply too much to bear.

So, I made a movie. I decided to expose the absolute unacceptable behavior our family experienced. The things I found out were so chilling I even went under-cover. This film would eventually become the HBO documentary Bleed Out, *seen by over fifteen million people. So many great things have happened since my mom's story came out. We have met thousands of patients and families just like ours, the esteemed Patient Safety Movement Foundation named a humanitarian award after my mom, and the prestigious LeapFrog Group named an entire school after her! The Judie Burrows Education Institute was launched in March 2022 in Washington DC.* Bleed Out *has become a driving catalyst for patient safety across the world and my mom would be so happy knowing that lives are being saved because of her courageous fight.*

Even the new CEO of the hospital system that injured my mom called to say that after twelve years, they would do the right thing. Then we never heard from him again.

I was grateful to have patient safety advocates Martie Hatlie, Tracy Granzyk, Greg Vass, and Soojin Jun joining me on my walk this morning. Before leaving American Family Fields, I led a memorial service for Judie Burrows, placing a yellow painted memorial stone with her name written on it in a small garden just outside the ballpark.

The first half of our route took us through the west side of Milwaukee—a city that seems to have stalled in the 1970s, leaving its architecture and infrastructure in need of a face lift. Almost every major street corner had a neighborhood tavern on the first floor of a 1950s two-story brick building. The popular '70s TV show *Laverne and Shirley* came to mind, the catchy musical intro accompanying Penny Marshall and Cindy Williams, skipping down the street to work as bottle cappers at the fictional Shotz Brewery. At each bar we passed, a Pabst, Hamm's, or Schlitz neon sign collector's item hung in the black-painted storefront window.

After walking sixteen miles, we arrived at Grant Park Plaza in South Milwaukee, where we ended day one. Steve and Margo were again waiting for us and were joined by Wisconsin Congresswoman Christine Sinicki. Being an avid supporter of patient safety, Christine has worked with Wisconsin families impacted by medical error. The congresswoman learned of Judie's story and reached out to the Burrows. She recently introduced three patient safety legislative bills for approval. One of the bills titled "Judie's Law," after Judie Burrows, would ensure that adult children are added to the list of relatives entitled to damages because of harm to or the death of a parent. A second bill, "The Julie Rubenzer Black Box Bill," if passed, would require any place where surgical procedures are performed to offer patients the option of having their procedures and discharge instructions videotaped. In the Judie Burrows case, when the time came for the surgeons, anesthesiologists, ICU nurses, and other staff to give their depositions under oath, care team members suddenly could not remember what happened in the operating room that day. When questioned during the depositions, they frequently responded with "I don't recall." The anesthesiologist could not recall if a second anesthesiologist was urgently called into the operating room to help, even though the surgeon had said a second anesthesiologist was indeed called in and was there in surgery for two or three hours. The ICU nurse could not remember changing Judie's medical record, even though the electronic medical record shows Judie's medical record was changed six times by the nurse during her ICU stay.

Aviation uses a flight recorder, known as a "black box," which records and preserves data from commercial airplanes that can be used later for learning purposes and safety improvement initiatives. The use of a black box in healthcare that records surgical procedures like Judie's can have similar safety benefits and would have answered questions that remain unanswered today because of the "I don't recall" legal defense strategy.

Monday, July 6th, 2020 (Day Two)

We had driven almost 2,000 miles since leaving Phoenix and done so without any major incidents along the way. Monday, July 6th, however, would test our reserves. We woke up to a one-inch round bubble on the side of the back right tire looking like it was ready to burst. During a normal holiday week, this would be a challenging impromptu task, but during a pandemic, it took hours from the coolest part of the day. After replacing the tire, we arrived back at Grant Park Plaza around 11:30am, where we were met by the local Fox TV news reporter who filmed the start of our walk as Cathy and I exited the parking lot. We were masked and social distanced from one another, when out of nowhere, a rusted-out, red Ford F150 pick-up truck screeched to a stop. Startled and scared, all three of us froze wondering what would happen next.

An older man, who looked to be in his sixties, jumped out of the driver's side and glared at us through half-closed, blood shot eyes. His face, wrinkled and weathered, looked like he had spent years baking in the sun. A lit cigarette hung from his bottom lip. He inhaled deeply before exhaling a large ring of smoke. Then he pulled the cigarette from his mouth, stomped it out on the ground with his boot heal and began screaming: "Take those damn stupid masks off right now!"

Cathy and I plus the reporter stood speechless, not wanting to provoke him anymore. He proceeded to the back of his truck, while pointing his index finger at us, repeating: "I said take those damn masks off right now!"

In a state of shock, I continued looking at him wondering how much worse this might get. For a brief moment, I thought he was going to walk over to the three of us on the sidewalk and physically pull our masks off. My heart was racing and my hands started trembling from the adrenaline surge now going through my body. It was clear he wanted to pick a fight about wearing masks in public. Was mask wearing now a sign of political allegiance: Democrats wear masks, and Republicans do not? Had choosing to wear or not wear a mask polarized our country to this extreme?

We remained silent, not wanting further confrontation.

"Fuck you!" He shouted before retreating back into his truck and peeling away.

I wondered to myself what might have happened if he did throw a punch at one of us, or worse, pulled a gun from under the seat of his truck, using the firearm to persuade us to remove our masks. My heart rate finally slowed as the three of us tried catching our breath before returning to the interview. The reporter was visibly shaken, laying his large shoulder-mounted TV camera on the ground before taking a deep breath, finally exhaling it a couple seconds later and now smiling again as color returned to his face. We had been heads-down in our mission and naïve to the extent of the polarization taking place across the country.

Just north of Racine, I came across the Hob Nob lounge and restaurant. The restaurant had a twenty-foot tall martini glass painted on the front of the two-story building. After our last confrontation, I felt like I could use a martini right now but fortunately the restaurant was closed. The restaurant and lounge had a retro '50s look, the type of place one would expect to hear Frank Sinatra, Dean Martin, Sammy Davis Jr., or Doris Day playing on the juke box. About a quarter of a mile later, I stopped and entered an old bowling alley right out of the 1950s, the bowling lanes still using manual pin-setting. The Hob Nob lounge and bowling alley made me feel like I was in the movie *Back to the Future* expecting Fonzie from *Happy Days* to walk out the front door. Wisconsin was again refusing to move forward into the new millennium, let alone 2020.

Tuesday, July 7th, 2020 (Day Three)

Walking through south Racine, WI, about twenty miles north of the Illinois border, posters supporting Black Lives Matter, the Rainbow Coalition, and American Unity hung in many of the storefront windows and were staked onto the manicured lawns in front of old Victorian homes and turn-of-the-century brick bungalows. Reaching Kenosha, everything changed. Gone were the sailboat-lined harbor, small-town boutiques, and quaint restaurants we loved in Racine. In the heart of Kenosha stood old, rundown, paint-peeling brick buildings in contrast to the brightly colored murals and coalition posters in Racine. There was a palpable tension in the air, people were less friendly, and there was no eye contact. Many of them looked angry. A nearby bank building with a neon sign on the burnt-out yellowing lawn flashed 97 degrees at 10:30am. A message followed, alerting residents and visitors of an excessive heat warning in place for the rest of the day, with humidity readings matching the air temperature.

A few weeks later, the tension we sensed exploded when on August 23rd a Kenosha police officer shot an unarmed Black man during a domestic disturbance, paralyzing him from the waist down, and spurring additional riots. Midwestern militia armed with rifles and automatic weapons arrived in the city, wanting to further fuel the chaos by inserting themselves into the riots that followed the protests. For three nights, the chaos continued, eventually ending when shots were fired, leaving two men dead and one more wounded.

Thursday July 9th, 2020 (Day Five)

We were on our way walking from Waukegan, Illinois, to Highwood, Illinois, the soaring temperatures and humidity levels staying with us. Abandoned factories and industrial buildings lined the road on both sides with peeling paint and broken windows sitting on rusted steel girders. The vacant fields nearby were littered with shredded car tires, bottles, cans, and other assorted debris. A couple miles later, we reached the northern suburb of Lake Bluff, now walking on well-cared-for bike trails and sidewalks, upon which in pre-pandemic days we'd have been dodging crowds of walkers and cyclists. It was as if we had crossed into a completely different country.

Saturday, July 11th, 2020 (Day Seven)

On our last day of the Chicago leg, I pulled my Ron Santo vintage 1969 Cubs jersey out of the hotel closet. I planned on wearing Santo's jersey weeks in advance, not only proving my wife's teasing to be warranted, but also because he is one of the greatest Chicago Cubs of all time. Santo, a Hall of Famer, played third base for the Cubs from 1960 to 1973, and became a popular Cubs radio broadcaster from 1990 until his death in 2010.

I was joined by friends and colleagues, who met Cathy and I on the Northwestern University campus where we parked our car to begin the walk. I was excited that Tim McDonald, a good friend, fellow anesthesiologist, patient safety partner, and national patient safety leader was walking with me today.

Arriving at Wrigley Field, FOX, ABC, and CBS local television stations were waiting for us, making my interview appear as breaking news or an important press conference. Each station had placed a microphone stand in front of me, and each reporter took turns asking me questions about my walk across America, about patient safety and preventable harm, and about my love of baseball and the Chicago Cubs.

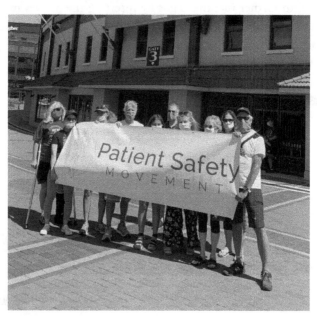

Team Picture
Photo courtesy of Dave Mayer (2020)

At the Ernie Banks statue, we did a memorial service with memorial stones for Michelle Ballog, who died from preventable medical harm while I was working at the University of Illinois Hospital in Chicago, and for her father Bob Malizzo, who along with his wife, Barb, had been national leaders in the patient safety movement since their daughter's unnecessary death. Bob recently passed away, or he would have been there too, and he was missed by all of us who knew him.

Completing another major portion of my walk across America in a place so close to my heart was more emotional than I had expected. Wrigley Field is where I went at age six to my first baseball game with my father, where I took our son Scott to his first baseball game at age four, and where my son and I took our grandson to his first baseball game at ten months of age. Having walked through this Wrigleyville neighborhood every decade of my life, these streets held memories of friendships and time well-spent with family. Casey Moran's upstairs bar, the live music at Cubby Bear, the large collection of sports memorabilia at Murphy's Bar—every restaurant or bar I passed triggered a well-lived moment from my past, bringing tears of joy to my eyes. This was my city and my baseball team, and I am certain the smile on my face was visible despite being hidden by my mask.

Over the last seven days, I had covered another ninety-two miles and had survived the Midwest heat and humidity, finishing at Wrigley Field with outstanding media coverage. My plan of walking to ballparks raising awareness about preventable medical harm was working. The media was hungry for something to report on besides the pandemic and the political polarity, and it was becoming apparent that my walk was providing a "feel-good" story during one of the most devastating years our country has gone through.

"A good mentor hopes you move on; a great mentor knows you will move on."

Leslie Higgins; Ted Lasso TV show

July 13th, 2020

Miles walked = 1,031
Steps = 2,581,080

"Jimenez into the wind-up, the pitch, swing and a miss. Strike two!"

Walking down the right field side of Comerica Park, home of the Detroit Tigers baseball team, the faint voice of an announcer stopped me in my tracks. Was someone calling the play-by-play for a baseball game? Was I dreaming?

I kept edging closer to the right field corner, trying to find where the voice was coming from. Were the Tiger announcers practicing their craft, trying to stay sharp for the upcoming shortened season, or was it a recording of a 2019 Tigers game coming from one of the bars across the street from the stadium?

"The count on Reyes now at two balls, two strikes."

At right field, through a ten-foot chain-link entrance gate, the scoreboard lit up with live game statistics in full view, showing #22 at bat, two outs in the bottom of the second, and the batter's count at two balls and two strikes—all this announced by the mystery voice.

"Reyes swings and hits a sharp ground ball to first, Cabrera fields the ball, and makes the short run to the bag for the unassisted out."

The Tigers were playing a split-squad, simulated baseball game inside the park. The ballplayers were practicing for opening day less than two weeks away. I kept walking around the stadium, searching for another gate where I might catch a glimpse of the action on the field, but like most stadiums, the game's activity was available to only those sitting in the stands. Still, the players were back and that was encouraging, promising, and exciting. I missed baseball so much over the last few months that I began dreaming about this very moment, sitting in Wrigley Field as the players exited the dugout, running to their positions eagerly waiting for the first pitch to be thrown—fans on their feet cheering, hot dog and beer vendors hustling up and down the aisles satisfying a fan's hunger or quenching another's thirst.

Maybe baseball would open back up to fans later this season. Was this a harbinger of change, something positive to look forward to? As a physician, I understood the seriousness of this fast-spreading disease that sometimes resulted in death, but I've always retained a certain amount of hope that life might get back to normal sooner than anticipated. The science of contagious and deadly viruses, how they mutate, and the length of time it would take to develop a vaccine and herd immunity told me it was unlikely, but my heart kept hoping both science and baseball would come out on top— no matter the odds.

An hour earlier, we had arrived in Detroit and parked our car in front of Comerica Park. My plan was to do a four-mile walk around the downtown area, Comerica Park, and Ford Field, home of the Detroit Lions. For a Monday morning, downtown Detroit was deserted with only an occasional car navigating empty neighborhood streets.

A fifteen-foot tiger statue, the color of snow, welcomed me. The concession stands lining the walkways were boarded up—no more vendors selling hot dogs, peanuts, or beer, as noted on the green wooden menus above sealed windows. No flocks of fans anywhere.

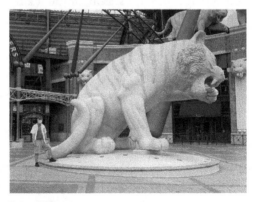

Detroit Tiger
Photo courtesy of Dave Mayer (2020)

Cathy and I walked around the park and we could see the familiar blue and silver signage of the Detroit Lions emblazoned on Ford Stadium three blocks away. A ghost town of sports bars and restaurants, once teeming with fans, lined both sides of the street between the two steel and red brick sports stadiums. All doors were locked tight.

After my four-mile walk, spending close to twenty minutes next to the right field gate listening to the radio announcer doing play-by-play for the simulated game, we headed to our next stop—Cleveland. Checking in at our hotel, we quickly changed into our walking clothes. I pulled my new Jason Kipnis Cubs jersey from the suitcase. Jason had been an all-star second baseman for the Cleveland Indians for nine years before signing a one-year contract to come back home to Chicago and play for the Cubs in 2020. Jason and his older brother Blair grew up in Northbrook and attended Glenbrook North High School with our children. It was Blair who introduced my son, Scott, to his wife, Leah, and all have remained close friends through the years. Watching a local kid make it to "The Show" as they say has added an extra element of investment to my fandom, and I was proud to wear his Cubs jersey in Cleveland.

Heading back down to the lobby of the hotel, we met national patient safety leader and advocate Chrissie Blackburn, the mother of a medically fragile thirteen-year-old daughter. Lily was born with an extremely rare disorder that resulted in several physical malformations requiring surgeries and follow-up visits. Chrissie has spent years navigating the health system on her daughter's behalf. Many times, Lily's care was good, but other times it was far from that. To Chrissie, the system was built for the benefit and ease of hospital administrators, physicians, and nurses, instead of the customers they serve—patients and families. Because of the inconsistencies in her daughter's treatment, Chrissie was always at Lily's bedside, taking notes and observing areas that could be improved. She joined committees at the University Hospitals Medical Center in Cleveland where her daughter received care and began contributing to improvement efforts, becoming a healthcare champion and agent of change. She wanted to help other patients and families learn how to partner with their care teams to achieve safe, high-quality care, and University Hospitals agreed. They hired her as the first Principal Advisor of Patient and Family Engagement, coaching patients and families on how to navigate the health care system. I was excited to have Chrissie, a nationally recognized leader in patient engagement, teamwork, and communication, joining me on my walk to the Cleveland Indians, now Guardians, Progressive Field.

Chrissie shared this passage about her daughter Lily with me:

Lily is the reason I do everything for patient safety. In addition to her life of being a beautiful, medically complex child, it is my passion and work to ensure all people receive the safest care. I have a long legacy of healthcare safety in my family. My mother taught me and my two older sisters how to speak up and how to form partnerships with providers and staff. This teaching gave me the confidence to speak up for Lily. I walked with Dr. Mayer to teach others to speak up in the healthcare setting. Although it may be scary at times to be a part of the care team, your voice is critically IMPORTANT. I stand by patient safety. It is imperative that we make it a priority for all of us that receive healthcare.

Chrissie, Cathy, and I walked down 9th Street to the ballpark, stepping over shards of broken glass crunching beneath our feet. Storefronts were boarded up with sheets of graffiti-covered plywood. Like other cities across the country, Cleveland had been hit hard by Black Lives Matter protests that erupted into nightly rioting, violence, and looting over the last few weeks. Local news programs had aired videos of rioters throwing rocks at police officers, reporting that ninety-nine people had been arrested on various counts ranging from curfew violations to assault and battery to resisting arrest. Our visit to Cleveland provided a firsthand view of the racism and hatred that had been escalating over the years, tearing our country apart. Less in the lens of current events were the increasing numbers of attacks on Jewish synagogues, cemeteries, monuments, and Jewish people that had been escalating at alarming rates over the last number of years.

After almost two miles of walking, four light towers above the right-field stands became visible on the opposite side of the street. The last time I walked down 9th Street to Progressive Field was on October 2nd, 2016, with my youngest daughter, Carlie, both of us just short of giddy heading into game seven of the 2016 World Series between the Chicago Cubs and Cleveland Indians.

Many baseball historians, as well as most Cubs fans, say game seven of the 2016 World Series was the greatest game seven in baseball history. The Cleveland Indians and the Chicago Cubs had not won a World Series in a collective 178 years, the Tribe going seventy years and the Cubs a painful 108 years—the two longest championship droughts in Major League Baseball. Baseball fans watching the game inside Progressive Field and across the country rode an emotional extra-inning rollercoaster watched by over forty million people on TV that evening.

After Dexter Fowler led off the game with a home run giving Chicago a 1–0 lead, Cubs fans in attendance were so loud, many watching on TV wondered if the game was being played in Wrigley Field. There was a sea of Cubby-blue attire everywhere. Some fans drove five hours from Chicago to Cleveland on I-90; others like Carlie and me flew using Southwest Airlines to punch our game seven tickets, while the corporate elite and star-studded celebrities sitting in the highest-priced seats landed in private jets. Box seat tickets around home plate for game seven on the open market sold for upwards of $25,000 per seat.

The Cubs continued to build their lead through the first seven innings. Leading 6–3 as the game entered the bottom of the eighth, Cubs fans bit their fingernails down to the knub knowing they had been here before. In 2003, with the Cubs up 3–1 and two outs in the top of the eighth inning, our lovable losers imploded against the Miami Marlins, eventually losing the game 8–3 and the National League Championship series the following day.

After two quick outs in the bottom of the eighth inning, Jose Ramirez singled. I turned my back to the infield in disgust.

"Carlie, I've seen this movie before," I shouted above the groans of other Cubs fans. "We're going to blow it. Always the same inning—always the eighth inning after two outs with only four outs to go."

"Think positive, Dad!" she countered, not having the gray hair or memories of six decades of losing like her father.

"I can't look," I replied, refusing to turn around and watch the next at bat.

Cleveland fans were on their feet, cheering and sensing a comeback. They too knew the Cubs history, the curse we could not shake, and the Cubs way of losing baseball games that appeared to be won.

"Why can't it be easy? Why can't they close out this game?" I was mumbling under my breath.

"Maddon's coming out to the mound, he's taking Lester out of the game," my daughter yelled into my ear. I turned around just as the Cubs manager raised his left arm, signaling Aroldis Chapman in the bull pen.

John Lester had been the Cubs' starting pitcher in games one and five but was called on to relieve Kyle Hendricks in the fifth inning, making his first relief appearance since 2007. There is no game eight in a World Series, so Maddon was doing whatever it might take to win game seven.

Chapman had already pitched in games five and six, and Maddon was asking him to hold Chicago's 6–3 lead, Cubs fans hoping Chapman had four more outs in his well-worn left arm. Our ace reliever's first few pitches to Brandon Guyer ended with an RBI double. I turned my back to the playing field again, the sinking feeling of "wait until next year" rising from the pit in my stomach. Standing face-to-face with worried Cubs fans sitting behind me along the first base line, the looks on their faces would make one believe a tornado was coming straight at us. Instead, I chose to cling to Carlie's "stay positive" vibe, and turned back around just as Rajai Davis, who had only hit fifty-five homers in eleven MLB seasons, golfed a low inside pitch for a home run that barely cleared the left field fence. Boom! The Cubs three-run lead was gone, the game tied at 6–6. Slumping into my chair with my hands over my head, I could not believe what we had just witnessed. The curse was back. It would never go away... not in my lifetime.

I was sick to my stomach and sat motionless. Cubs and Indians fans sat through a scoreless ninth, sending the game into extra innings. Suddenly, and only in true Cubs dramatic fashion, the warm and humid November skies opened up, soaking players and fans during the infamous seventeen-minute rain delay. Cubs fans in our section sat bewildered and shell-shocked in our seats, too numb to seek cover from the rain. None of us were aware that Jason Heyward, the Cubs right fielder, had called a team meeting in the visitor's weight room during the short rain delay. It was the first team meeting called by the players all year. By most accounts, Heyward gave a charged pep talk to his teammates, reminding them that they were the best team in the League and that this game was theirs to win, not lose. Re-energized, the Cubs picked up their bats to start the tenth inning.

Kyle Schwarber, only recently back in the lineup after a season-ending knee injury in April, led off the tenth inning with a single just out of reach of Jason Kipnis at second base. I was now back on my feet in my wet Cubs jersey, trying to shake off the desperation of the last hour.

"There we go!" I said to my daughter, high-fiving her and the other surrounding Cubs fans.

Albert Almora, who came in to run for Schwarber, tagged up and reached second on a deep fly ball. Cubs fans began chanting "Go Cubs Go" once again, all of us trying to forget the pain of the eighth inning.

Anthony Rizzo was intentionally walked before game MVP, Ben Zobrist, delivered an RBI double just out of reach of Cleveland's diving third baseman.

With the Cubs up 7–6, the rollercoaster of emotions shifted between the two fan bases yet again. Cubs fans were back on their feet, screaming and hugging each other; Cleveland fans were back in their seats, annoyed by the overzealous Cubs fans jumping up and down around them. The Cubs added one more run in the top of the tenth inning, giving them an 8–6 lead heading into the bottom of the tenth.

Carlie and I began chanting "Three more outs," then "Two more outs," and finally "One more out" with others around us as the first two Cleveland hitters were retired by Carl Edwards Jr. The Tribe added a run after two consecutive hits, making it 8–7, but for some reason this momentum shift felt different. We were past the cursed eighth inning and like our team on the field, fans also felt re-energized. I was not waiting for dreadful things to happen like in the eighth inning. I was thinking positive things were ahead for Cubs fans, like my daughter told me they would be.

With the tying run on first base and the winning run standing at home plate for the Indians, Cubs reliever Mike Montgomery, with zero career saves in his professional career to that point, forced Michael Martinez to hit a weak ground ball, which third-baseman Kris Bryant charged, scooped, and threw to Rizzo at first base. Rizzo waving his glove in joyous victory before tucking the ball into his back pocket is a moment in Cubs history seared in my memory. It had taken four hours and twenty-eight minutes for the Chicago Cubs to earn their first World Series championship title in 108 years and about every minute of that game was electric.

Four years later, I was at the same center field entrance to the stadium. Chrissie, Cathy, and I walked around to the home plate entrance where we met a local news reporter and film crew. They interviewed Chrissie and me about what we were doing here and why. The reporter loved my Kipnis jersey and joked about the danger of wearing it in Cleveland, where fans were unhappy the team had released him during the off-season, especially to the Chicago Cubs.

As we rounded the left field corner and headed up the concrete walkway leading back toward centerfield, I saw local fans—people wearing Cleveland Indians jerseys standing and cheering in front of the left field gate. I approached the chain-link fence and saw ballplayers taking batting practice swings inside the park. Then, I heard one of my favorite sports-related sounds: the crack of a wood bat against a baseball at the thickest point, the sweet spot of the wood. It's a sound all baseball fans love, especially when watching a hometown favorite connect with a fastball to send it out of the park for a homerun. Crack! I heard it again, this time pulling out my cell phone and recording the sound for enjoyment later. Then, just as the reporter predicted, a few Cleveland fans spotted my Cubs Kipnis jersey and the taunts began. "Kipnis will always be a Cleveland Indian," one fan shouted. "Number 22 looked so much better on him than your Number 27," one fan chided, referring to the number Jason now wears with the Cubs and that I had on my back. I took the ribbing well, having been a Chicago sports fan all my life and knowing that riling up the hometown crowd was never a good idea. After ten minutes, the three of us headed back to the hotel where we completed our four-mile walk for the day.

"We must accept that human error is inevitable—and design
around that fact."

Dr. Donald Berwick

The next morning, Cathy and I were back on the road, driving to Pittsburgh to walk to the Pirates' PNC Park. With Cathy behind the wheel, I was able to squeeze in a phone interview with Joshua Axelrod, a reporter for the *Pittsburgh Post-Gazette*. Josh is a sportswriter with a deep knowledge of baseball and its history. We shared stories about the 1979 Pittsburgh Pirates team that won the World Series with Willie Stargell and Dave Parker leading the way. That team adopted the Sister Sledge hit song, "We are Family," and played it at every home game that season. I shared one of few Cubs playoff memories— watching Harry Caray call the 1984 Chicago Cubs game when they clinched a playoff berth in Pittsburgh for the first time since 1945 with manager Jim Frey at the helm. Starting pitcher Rick Sutcliffe pitched a complete game gem, giving up two hits that night and striking out the final Pirate batter for a 4–1 win. Another Cubs memory planted in my brain is the entire team rushing out of the dugout to celebrate Sutcliffe on the mound. Like the Pirates, the Cubs had adopted their own song that special season, "Jump" by Van Halen, and it fit at least until their only post-season play since 1945 ended in a 3–2 series loss to the San Diego Padres.

I love baseball because of its leisurely pace. It's different from other team sports. The high-energy and physical contact found in football, basketball, and hockey fires me up, but that's not always what I need. Instead of blocking and tackling in football, fighting for rebounds in basketball, or checking an opponent into the boards in hockey, baseball is an acrobatic shortstop diving into the outfield to snag a ground ball, then leaping and turning in mid-air like a ballerina while firing the ball to first base for the out. It's an athletic centerfielder crashing against the wall to rob a hitter of a home run. Baseball is ballet and dance compared to hand-to-hand combat of other team sports. Ted Williams once said, "The hardest thing to do in baseball is to hit a round baseball with a round bat, squarely."

Some people think baseball needs to speed up, less time between pitches, limiting trips by managers to the mound and stopping batters from stepping out of the batter's box. I disagree. My four hours of peaceful bliss is sitting on a molded green plastic seat under a majestic blue sky at Wrigley Field. The experience isn't complete without sipping an ice-cold 312 pale ale beer, eating a Chicago-style Vienna hot dog with mustard (never ketchup), and catching a bag of salted-in-the-shell peanuts purchased from a vendor in a blue jersey who throws a strike every time after yelling, "Peanuts here, roasted peanuts!" That's what excites me.

As a cardiac anesthesiologist, the slower pace of baseball was important for me. My world consisted of a non-ending string of high-stress cardiac surgical cases—newborn babies with congenital complexities, seriously ill patients requiring lung or heart transplants, people dying in front of our eyes as we rushed them to the operating room for bypass surgery. I loved every moment of my professional career, but I also needed the quiet "recharging" periods baseball provided for my own mental well-being. Baseball, more than any sport, allowed me to "check out," to enjoy four hours of competitive action while turning the rest of the world off.

Once again, I decided to wear my Joe Maddon Cubs jersey while walking around PNC Park. Maddon had grown up in Hazelton, Pennsylvania, a town of 25,000 people in northwest Pennsylvania and he maintains close roots with the town with his charity work, helping start the Hazelton Integration Project. Teaching all generations about diversity and acceptance, the Hazelton Integration Project works to unite people from different cultural backgrounds. Its community center offers programs that support hundreds of local residents each week.

I walked around the ballpark while being interviewed by local ABC and CBS television reporters and was struck by the beauty of the ballpark built upon the banks of the Allegheny River across from the downtown Pittsburgh skyline. The design had an intentional "retro" feel, reminding me of Wrigley Field with its classic architecture, natural grass surface, and outstanding sight lines. Twelve-foot-tall bronze statues of Hall of Famers Willie Stargell, Roberto Clemente, Bill Mazeroski, and Honus Wagner were placed individually one on each side of the ballpark welcoming fans to the stadium.

But it was the colorful twenty-foot banners hanging from steel posts jutting out from the stadium's limestone façade that left a lasting impression in our minds. Each banner had a large photo of a local healthcare worker. This was the Pirates' way of celebrating these courageous men and women working on the frontlines during the pandemic. The banners expressed gratitude from the team for the heroism of a particular healthcare worker pictured above in a life-size photo. Both Cathy and I were emotionally moved by this touching tribute to those risking their lives every day while doing what they love—caring for patients.

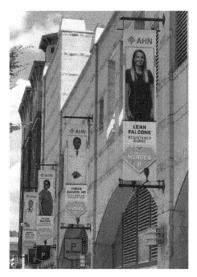

PNC Park
Photo courtesy of Dave Mayer (2020)

Taking care of hospitalized patients has been steeped in potential pitfalls for both patients and providers since long before the pandemic began. Despite the attempt at building safe care environments, healthcare workers suffer numerous work-related injuries such as needle sticks, lifting and back injuries, falls with debilitating injuries, and increased workplace violence ranging from verbal abuse to criminal assaults—all contributing to high instances of burnout, depression, and suicide, only to be compounded by demands in the environment created by the spread of COVID-19.

Since the start of the pandemic, the safety of every healthcare professional from environmental services to respiratory therapists to EMTs, nurses, and physicians has been in jeopardy. In the first four months, hundreds lost their lives because of COVID-19. More healthcare workers became infected, requiring hospitalization including admission to intensive care units for days, weeks, and some even months. Public health experts believe many of these early deaths and hospitalizations would have been preventable if we had been better prepared by having adequate policy and pandemic training in place, or if our supply-chain management leaders had considered the potential for shortages of protective equipment (gowns, gloves, and masks), diagnostic tests, and ventilators.

Between 2019 and 2020, workplace violence rates tripled in one Missouri hospital, leading leadership to install a panic button system on staff members badges.[7] A study published in 2021 by Byon et al. reported that 44.4 percent of nurses experienced physical violence and 67.8 percent experienced verbal abuse between February 2020 and June 2020, the first few months of the pandemic.[8] AP news reported that doctors and nurses in Idaho feared for their lives because family members who didn't believe in COVID-19 were accusing them of killing their loved ones. Because of misinformation spread over social media, healthcare workers were scared to be out in public, fearing personal attacks against them.[9]

An August 6th, 2021, study using thousands of nurses across the country, published by Morgan Curry, BSN, RN and Nursing CE Central, found that 95 percent of the nurses reported feeling burned out in their nursing positions over the last three years, with 49.7 percent looking for less-stressful nursing positions, or having left nursing all-together because of the burnout.[10]

The deaths, and the growing number of psychosocial and behavioral health needs of our workforce, were daunting to think about. Back in the

[7] Shivaram, Deepa. A Hospital Gives Its Staff Panic Buttons After Assaults By Patients Triple. www.Npr.org. September 30th, 2021.

[8] Byon HD, Sagherian K, Kim Y, Lipscomb J, Crandall M, Steege L.Workplace Health Saf. 2021 Aug 3:21650799211031233. doi: 10.1177/21650799211031233. Online ahead of print.PMID: 34344236

[9] Boone, Rebecca. Misinformation Leads to animosity towards health care workers. www. apnews.com. September 29th, 2021.

[10] Curry, Morgan. Nursing CE Central: Nurse Burnout Study 2021. www.nursingcecentral. com. August 6th, 2021.

hotel that evening, I opened my computer and came across a story written by Gabriella Borter at Reuters, who covered the suicide of William Coddington, a thirty-two-year-old nurse in Florida who became upset watching patients his age die from the virus. Nursing was his dream job, and he was committed to his ten-year recovery from opioid addiction and substance abuse. Family and friends told Borter of his fears surrounding a lack of proper protective gear and that he suffered from nightmares about ventilator alarms going off in the ICU. Coddington was found dead in his car, a family member suspecting he died from a drug overdose, having been unable to attend his twelve-step program meetings in person during quarantine.

I also returned to the "Lost on the Front Lines" website and chose two healthcare workers who died because of COVID-19 and dedicated my walk in Pittsburgh and PNC Park in memory of both on social media (#Walk-ForPTSafety). Here are their stories:

Bernard Etta was a sixty-one-year-old registered nurse who worked in the Ohio prison system. As COVID hit Ohio, family members urged Bernard to stop working, concerned he wouldn't have the protective gear needed to keep him safe. Citing his duty to work and the belief there was adequate protection, he continued to work long hours. Bernard started having symptoms and tested positive for COVID, staying at home, fearing the cost of hospital bills. He died on May 17th, 2020, leaving behind a wife, four children, and several grandchildren.[11]

Sean Boynes was a forty-six-year-old pharmacist from Maryland. When COVID started hitting the Washington, DC region, he continued to go to work, telling family that patients needed their medications. Sean was a Howard University Alumnus, having three different degrees from the university including a master's in exercise physiology and a doctorate in pharmacy. In early March, Sean began feeling sick but didn't want to stop working. Finally taking a sick day, Sean's history of asthma added to his difficulties breathing. On March 25th, his wife dropped him at the hospital doors. His family including two small children, never saw him again. To honor Sean, the pharmacy where he worked was named after him.[12]

---

[11] "Lost on the Frontline". KHN.org. Kaiser Health News and The Guardian. August 10,2020.
[12] "Lost on the Frontline". KHN.org. Kaiser Health News and The Guardian. August 10,2020.

The next morning, I learned from a colleague that Dr. John Piano, the surgical resident who paged me at 2:00am letting me know about Mr. Sandoval, our septic kidney stone patient who almost died on the operating table that night because my supervising attending decided to go back to sleep leaving me by myself, died a few days before from COVID-19. John's death and the deaths of other caregivers only fueled my passion and the need to continue raising awareness about problems I knew that would only get worse if not pushed into the spotlight.

Today, I walked in memory of Dr. Piano.

"No human race is superior; no religious faith is inferior. All collective judgments are wrong. Only racists make them."

Elie Wiesel

July 18th, 2020

Miles walked = 1,054
Steps = 2,629,820

On Monday, July 18th, Cathy and I arrived in Columbia, Maryland, for my long walks in Baltimore and Washington DC. We had been on the road for over a month, adding over 2,700 miles to our tired Audi camper.

It had been months since I was last in Maryland, the pandemic having changed the way we all lived and worked. Instead, my team and I met daily using cell phones, Zoom, and other virtual video platforms. Being virtual was painful, everyone spending half the meeting informing others they were still on mute. The pandemic had reduced family time with our children and grandchildren. It also deprived me of personal interactions with friends and coworkers. I was frustrated and depressed, wanting the virus to vanish, and for my life to return to the way it was in 2019.

I walk daily to ease my frustrations and depression. Walking empowers me to remove myself from a series of interiors disconnecting us from each other. While I'm on my feet, everything stays connected. It allows me to live in the whole world, rather than in spaces built up against it. Walking is the way to meaning, giving us a clearer vision of what's to come. All of this is from the simple act of placing one foot in front of the other. And I'm conscious and thankful each day for my ability to walk the landscape in whatever city I'm visiting or living.

My dear friends Jack and Teresa Gentry wanted to be part of my Maryland walk. Jack spent thirty-seven years working as a Baltimore police officer, the last seventeen of those years on the SWAT team as a skilled negotiator. Teresa worked as a nurse for forty-one years. Their lives changed dramatically in April of 2013 when a medical error occurred during spine surgery that left Jack paralyzed from the neck down. Unlike Steve and Margo Burrow's experience with their mother, Judie, the surgeon and hospital were transparent with the Gentrys and apologized for the life-changing, catastrophic event. MedStar Health covered the costs for Jack's surgery, the five months of rehabilitation, and other long-term needs such as renovations for their home and a wheelchair-accessible van. As a result of the open, honest, and compassionate approach used by MedStar, Jack and Teresa went on to become national advocates for honesty and transparency after preventable medical harm, traveling across the country sharing their story with leading healthcare systems.

Jack and Teresa wanted to be a part of my walk across America and came up with an idea to join us at Ripken Stadium. Jack felt the Baltimore walk to Camden yards would be difficult for him trying to navigate the streets and paths with his wheelchair.

Ripken Stadium is home to the Baltimore Orioles' class-A minor league team, the Ironbirds, and hosts many youth baseball tournaments during the year. The ballpark is about twenty minutes from their home.

The Gentrys had become close friends with others who suffered catastrophic, preventable losses such as Carole Hemmelgarn, Steve and Margo Burrows, and Bob and Barb Malizzo. They all belong to a special club no one wants to be a member of.

"Great idea, Jack! Did Teresa give her approval?" I knew who the boss was in their household, Teresa always keeping Jack from pushing himself too hard.

"Full approval, Dave. She is also excited about the idea."

Knowing Teresa was on board, I replied, "It would mean the world to me if you and Teresa could join me. Let's do it!"

On Sunday, July 24th at 7:30am, Cathy and I met Jack and Teresa at Ripken Stadium. Jack rode in his wheelchair as Teresa, Cathy, and I walked around the ballpark. It was a hot and steamy day. Beads of sweat rolled down our foreheads like condensation on a pitcher of cold lemonade.

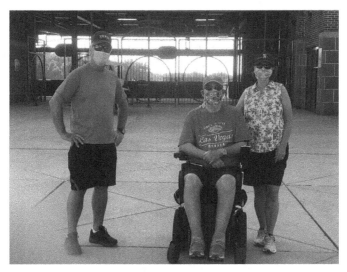

Teresa and Jack Gentry with the author
Photo courtesy of Dave Mayer (2020)

We stopped to watch youth baseball games being played on the eight different fields, each being a replica of a Major League ballpark. The parents sitting in the stands weren't wearing masks or social distancing. The umpires at home plate stood ten feet to the side of the plate, wearing masks and making vain attempts at calling balls and strikes.

All our shirts were completely soaked from perspiration after the four miles, but no one complained. The twinkle in Jack's and Teresa's eyes at the end of the walk was inspiring.

Day one of my two-day, twenty-two-mile walk to Camden Yards started on Friday, July 24th at the MedStar Health corporate office building and would finish at the Maryland Patient Safety Center (MPSC) offices, where I served as board chairman. Katie Carlin and Crystal Morales, two of my MedStar Health teammates, were walking with us today. A *Baltimore Sun* newspaper photographer met us for the last three miles of our walk, interviewing the four of us, while taking pictures for the article. After a three-month delay, Major League Baseball was returning that weekend albeit without fans in the ballparks, so baseball was back in the news.

A small crowd of people from the MPSC were there to welcome us after completing eleven miles. Everyone joined us for our memorial rock ceremony and moment of silence for Pat Sheridan, the husband of my friend and inter-nationally recognized patient safety advocate Sue Sheridan. Pat grew up in Baltimore and was an avid Orioles fan; his favorite player was Cal Ripken, Jr., nicknamed the "Iron Man" for playing in 2,632 straight games, a Major League Baseball record. Never having had the opportunity to meet Pat before his unfortunate death, I had no doubt we would have bonded through our mutual love of baseball.

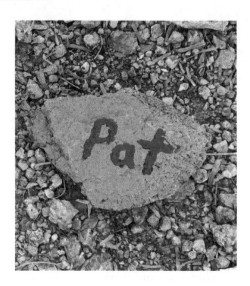

Sue Sheridan shared the following passage about her husband Patrick with me.

My husband Patrick Sheridan, Global Division Manager for a software company and father of two young children, began to develop pain in his neck and shoulders. Although he sought out physical therapy and then acupuncture as ordered by his primary care doctor, the pain persisted. An orthopedic specialist finally ordered an MRI scan that revealed a concerning mass in his cervical spine.

Pat was referred to a well-respected teaching hospital in another state where a neurosurgeon successfully removed the mass. Based on the preliminary pathology report, the surgeon reassured Patrick and his wife, Sue, that it was a benign tumor and that he did not need further treatment.

Over the next few weeks additional tests were performed on the specimen, resulting in a final pathology report that was faxed to Patrick's neurosurgeon.

Apparently, the final pathology report was filed in Patrick's medical record without the neurosurgeon ever seeing it. No action was taken.

Our family celebrated what they thought was his recovery. Six months later, the pain was back. The lost pathology report was now discovered. The final diagnosis turned out to be an aggressive, malignant sarcoma requiring urgent treatment.

During the six months of non-treatment, the tumor metastasized and penetrated his spinal cord. Patrick endured seven additional surgeries and several rounds of chemotherapy and radiation, but the cancer persisted. At the end of Patrick's life, he was paralyzed from the neck down. He died in 2002 when he was forty-five years old.

Patrick Sheridan's death is just one of an estimated 80,000 diagnostic errors that occur in health care each year. Some diagnostic errors do not lead to patient harm, but too many others cause permanent harm or death. Communication breakdowns between caregivers and standard follow-up of critical test results deprived Pat of the immediate treatment that could have saved his life. Instead, the medical error allowed the cancer to spread in his body over a six-month period, depriving him and his family of that possibility.

On Saturday morning, Cathy and I drove to west Canton, a historic community located on Baltimore's Inner Harbor. Wearing a Baltimore Orioles jersey, my walking route took us along the inner harbor boardwalk, over the cobblestone streets of Fells Point, through the restaurant district in Harbor East, and past the Pier Six outdoor concert venue, COVID having caused the cancellation of their entire 2020 season. Moving inland, we walked through the Federal Hill district, passing 200-year-old red-brick homes and buildings before ascending the stairway to the top of Federal Hill that overlooks the harbor where we could see Fort Henry. The failure of the British Navy to overtake the fort in 1814 was the inspiration for "The Star Spangled Banner" written by Francis Scott Key, who saw the U.S. flag proudly waving over the fort when he awoke the following morning.

Arriving at the east side of Camden Yards, Jack and Teresa Gentry were there to meet us, along with an NPR reporter and local TV crew who filmed our memorial stone service in memory of Louise Batz, the mother of good friend and national patient safety leader, Laura Batz Townsend, who founded the Louise H. Batz Patient Safety Foundation.

Louise Batz was a beloved wife, mother, sister, and grandmother who could light up a room with her beautiful smile and radiant glow. She was filled with love and brought happiness to both friends and strangers she would meet. Her needless death is another painful example of preventable medical harm.

Laura Batz Townsend shared this passage about her mother with me:

On April 14, 2009, my mom made the decision to have total knee-replacement surgery, battling a bum knee for greater than ten years. She had three grandchildren and one more on the way that she wanted to keep up with. We all felt comfortable and confident with her surgery, having five doctors in our family and a part of the San Antonio medical community for over 50 years.

The surgery was a success! The doctor was pleased with her new knee and said that she was ready to start the recovery process. The finish line was in sight! We sat with her all day and at 10:00pm, we were told to go home. I never imagined that would be the last time my mom would speak to me or tell me goodnight and that she loved me. I will forever wish that I had not gone home and stayed with her that night.

The phone rang around 3:15am. It was the hospital informing my dad that Mom was having trouble breathing. Racing to the hospital, I ran to her room, and at that moment I felt a pain that I have never experienced in my life. My mom was white, pale, lying still on the bed, and wasn't breathing on her own.

They told us my mom had suffered respiratory depression. The nurse had given her a nausea medication, morphine, and Meperidine at midnight but never went back to check on her.

My mom was on life support for ten days. During those days in the hospital, we asked questions about how this happened. It didn't take long before we realized she was in this condition because of a preventable medical mistake. How could this have happened?

I wondered if we were unlucky or if these types of errors occur with other patients. After doing research on medical errors, I learned that an estimated 250,000 people die every year from preventable medical harm, making it the third leading cause of death in the United States behind heart disease and cancer.

How did a family of doctors not know this or ever talk about it?

I told her how much I loved her and what a wonderful mother she was. I kept hoping for a miracle. Hoping that she would wake up, look at me, and assure me everything was going to be fine. But the damage to Mom's brain was too massive, and eight days later we were told that she would never recover. We made the painful decision to turn off life support. I sat with her until her heart "flat-lined."

Eleven days after her knee surgery, Mom died. She didn't die from a terminal illness or serious medical condition; she died from a preventable mistake.

From that moment on, I had a new sense of purpose and focus. My life took a different direction. I got up the next morning and wrote the mission and objectives of the Louise H. Batz Patient Safety Foundation. I was not going to let Mom's death go unnoticed. I couldn't imagine other families having to experience this pain.

If families work together with nurses and doctors as a team, these unfortunate outcomes would be different. Mom's death did not lie on the shoulders of one person; it was a team failure.

People come up to me and say all the time, "The one thing I remember most about your mom was her smile." It is so true. She had this amazing smile filled with love, happiness, and hope. It would literally light up a room. She was a wonderful friend, sister, grandmother, wife, and the best mom in the world.

She taught me how to love, respect, and care for others. To never give up, to always persevere, and most importantly never to lose hope. She was my hero. She saved my life every day and still does. I hope her story and legacy will inspire the hero in all of us.

I wish that I could have those five hours back.

As in Louise Batz's case, and many others who also have died from opioid-induced respiratory depression, potent opioid analgesics used for pain management can depress ventilation, potentially leading to serious morbidity and mortality. According to the Patient Safety Movement Foundation's website, over 50 percent of patients in the hospital receive opioids at some point in their care and of those patients, between 0.003 percent and 4.2 percent will experience an opioid-related adverse event between hospitalization and post-discharge, contributing to a 55 percent longer length of stay, 47 percent higher costs, 36 percent increased risk of readmission after 30 days, and 3.4 times greater likelihood of mortality. It is estimated that the majority of opioid-induced respiratory depression events within twenty-four hours of surgery could be prevented with better patient monitoring. Examples of monitors used to detect respiratory depression and decrease preventable harm from opioids include pulse oximetry and capnography.

July 28th, 2020. Washington DC.

Crossing the Potomac River heading south into Arlington, Virginia, one cannot but be moved by the site of thousands of white tombstones, perfectly lined in rows on the dark green grass rising up the hill. Arlington National Cemetery spans over 600 acres and is the final resting place of almost 400,000 who served our country and protected our freedom. I couldn't think of a better starting point for my walk to National Park, home of the Washington Nationals baseball team, wanting to remember those buried in the cemetery with a memorial rock ceremony at the baseball stadium.

On Tuesday morning, July 28th, Cathy, and I met Leah Binder, CEO of the LeapFrog Group, and Raj Ratwani, the director of the National Center for Human Factors Engineering in Healthcare at the entrance of the Arlington National Cemetery. Both are amazing people who have dedicated their lives to making care safer for others.

As their CEO for fourteen years, Leah Binder has been one of the nation's leaders in striving for safe, high-quality care for everyone. The LeapFrog Group publishes data on safety and quality outcomes, empowering people with the information they need to make better decisions about their health care. Founded twenty years ago by major U.S. corporations fed up with poor-quality health care, high preventable medical harm events, and growing costs, the LeapFrog Group uses an annual Hospital Rating System to publish grades for hospitals (A, B, C, D, or F) based on their safety and quality outcomes. The hospital grades allow consumers and purchasers of health care to educate themselves on the level of safety and quality of care provided by hospitals in their community. Dr. Ratwani is a nationally recognized human-factors scientist and expert who identifies system and process weaknesses in healthcare. His cutting-edge research has led to improvements in health care that save patient lives. I was honored to have both joining me this morning.

Crossing the Potomac River at the Arlington Memorial Bridge, we walked past the Lincoln Memorial before coming to the White House. Like many of the ballparks I had already visited, trying to find an opening where I could see inside the stadium, I struggled to find an opening in the newly constructed thirteen-foot fence and anti-climb walls to see the most famous residence in the country. Frustrated, I continued walking past a deserted Freedom Plaza before heading down a quiet Pennsylvania Avenue, only a scattering of cars or taxis driving on the normally crowded street to the Capitol Building. Circling back, Cathy and I walked down the mall to the Washington Monument before heading east on 14th Street SW toward National Park.

From fifty feet away, I felt the energy of a laser-focused gaze coming from a muscular six-foot, four-inch security guard in full uniform, a large black cap with a shiny brim keeping his head shaded from the sun. He looked me over from head to toe like a CT scanner as I approached the entrance of the United States Holocaust Memorial Museum. Like most tourist attractions in Washington DC, the pandemic had necessitated the closure of the museum. I peered through the glass entrance doors, looking to see if anyone might be inside, when I was startled by the deep voice of the security officer now standing a few feet behind me.

"Can I help you, sir?" his direct tone making me believe he had spent time in the military.

"Good morning," I responded, trying to ease his concerns about my intentions. In a single year, swastikas were sprayed or glued onto the Florida Holocaust Museum, the Alaska Jewish Museum, and the Oregon Holocaust Memorial. At the Sherwin Miller Museum of Jewish Art in Tulsa, Oklahoma, five statues dedicated to Jewish children killed during the Holocaust were destroyed, and the Washington DC Holocaust Museum has been a target of planned attacks including the fatal shooting of a museum security officer while on duty.

"I was out walking and wanted to stop by the museum, even though I knew it was closed," I told him, hoping he would relax. "I visited the museum many times before."

"Well, welcome back sir. Sorry you cannot go inside," he said, his voice softer now as he stepped back to the curb, his eyes continuing to alternate between watching me and looking up and down the street for the next possible attacker.

Standing quietly at the entrance, I reflected about the last ten days in Baltimore and Washington DC, meeting with good friends while walking to Camden Yards and National Park. They were memorable days but walking to the Holocaust Museum today had become the focal point of my time in the mid-Atlantic area. Walking 1,110 miles over the last five months gave me time to reflect about the Black Lives Matter protests and the escalating antisemitism occurring around the world. The museum was another reminder of that antisemitism, created so we never forget the systematic mass extermination of six million Jews, more than a third of the world's Jewish population at the time.

Growing up in Skokie, I felt protected from the antisemitism other Jews faced. It wasn't until I went to college that I found myself in the crosshairs of Jewish hatred from a few narrow-minded students. I joined a Jewish fraternity, Zeta Beta Tau (ZBT), one of three Jewish fraternities on campus. Over 75 percent of the pledges and brothers in these houses came from the northern suburbs of Chicago such as Skokie, Deerfield, and Highland Park. The remainder were from the western and southern suburbs of Chicago, except for the rare exception of a downstate Jew. A number of the non-Jewish fraternities referred to us as the "Kike" houses, an insulting, contemptuous term for a Jewish person that only fueled antisemitic views, actions, and hatred. It was clear that some non-Jewish fraternities disliked our houses simply because we were Jewish. Their bigotry had an energy of its own, coming to life during intramural football or basketball games between houses where cheap shots, intimidation, and confrontations seemed to occur more frequently than touchdowns or baskets. These opponents didn't just want to beat us, they wanted to hurt us.

As Elie Wiesel, a well-known author, Nobel Laureate, and Holocaust survivor said "To forget the dead would be akin to killing them a second time."

I vowed never to forget. After wiping tears from my eyes, I continued on to National Park where this emotional day would end, completing my nine-mile walk to National Park where two local TV station crews were waiting.

Packing our car that evening, we would now head south to Atlanta, Tampa Bay, and Miami, the nation's current COVID-19 hotbed.

"How old would you be if you didn't know how old you are?"

Satchel Paige
Hall of Fame pitcher who played his last MLB game
at the age of fifty-nine.

Wednesday, July 29th, 2020

Total Miles Walked = 1,119
Total Steps = 2,775,426

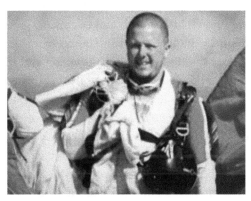

Joshua Nahum
Photo courtesy of Armando and Victoria Nahum

Joshua Nahum was an incredible, extremely bright, handsome twenty-seven-year-old man who absolutely adored children. No matter where he was, people gravitated to him as if he had a magnet that attracted the young and the old. And, wow, could he tell a story. Josh was preparing to become a child psychologist when he lost his life to preventable harm.

I cannot imagine what it is like to lose a child. My mind cannot even process such a thought without blocking it out, turning it off, changing the channel. With three children of my own, it's a subject I've never felt comfortable thinking about.

Those thoughts continued to haunt me during our nine-hour drive from Columbia, Maryland, to Atlanta, Georgia, where I would be meeting Armando Nahum, who would be walking with me today. Armando and his wife, Victoria, live in Atlanta and have dedicated their lives to raising awareness about sepsis and its early warning signs. The Nahum's lost their twenty-seven-year-old son Josh because early warning signs of sepsis were missed, causing delays in treatment that should have saved his life.

The Sepsis Alliance is the leading sepsis organization in the United States, raising awareness in all fifty states about the illness, its early warning signs and symptoms, and its treatments. According to their website, "Sepsis is the body's overwhelming and life-threatening response to infection that can lead to tissue damage, organ failure, and death. It's your body's overactive and toxic response to an infection. Like strokes or heart attacks, sepsis is a medical emergency that requires rapid diagnosis and treatment."

Every two minutes, someone in the United States dies of sepsis; the majority of sepsis cases start at home. Early detection and treatment of sepsis is critical. Signs and symptoms include a combination of any of the following: (1) confusion or disorientation, (2) shortness of breath, (3) high heart rate, (4) fever, shivering, or feeling very cold, (5) extreme pain or discomfort, and (6) clammy or sweaty skin. These signs and symptoms need to be taken seriously.

We arrived at Truist Field, home of the Atlanta Braves just before 4:00pm. Armando, dressed in beige shorts, a white T-shirt, and walking shoes, was standing next to his car in the hotel parking lot with his mask on, waiting for us. Cathy and I noticed a short, elderly woman in exercise clothes, also wearing a face mask standing next to Armando.

"Dave and Cathy, I would like to introduce my mother, Angela," Armando proclaimed.

"Mom asked if she could walk with us today in memory of Josh. She is eighty-seven-years old and walks two to three miles every morning to stay in shape."

It was clear her health plan was working, I thought, hoping I looked as good as she does when I'm in my eighties.

Angela chimed in. "I didn't walk this morning because I wanted to save my energy to walk with all of you."

The plan was to walk four miles around the ballpark and surrounding neighborhood. Truist Park, located ten miles west of downtown Atlanta in the community of Cumberland, is in an area known as The Battery Atlanta with its assortment of hotels, restaurants, and sports bars.

"Unfortunately, it's much warmer this afternoon than it probably was in the morning." I forewarned, giving anyone planning to walk a clear out.

Without hesitancy, Angela replied, "I am up for it! Lead the way."

As we began walking, all of us wearing masks and staying a safe distance from each other, Armando and Angela wanted to know more about my walk across America, the ballparks we visited, and the people who walked with us in those cities. As we chatted, I counted six hotels in the neighborhood, the largest being the Omni Hotel Atlanta Battery along the right field side of the ballpark, many of their rooms offering views of the baseball diamond. Nearing Truist Field, a couple hundred fans were congregating in the open-air restaurants and bars surrounding the ballpark.

A large neon marquee sign on the side of the ballpark caught my attention, making me chuckle under my mask.

"Welcome to the Atlanta Braves Home Opener" flashed in red lights. A message displayed for hundreds of fans enjoying their happy hour cocktails in the local restaurants and bars across the street to see, despite the fact fans were not allowed into the ballpark for the game.

We continued our walk, our shirts soaked from sweat, beads of perspiration falling off our noses, and baseball caps pulled down to protect us from the grueling sun. We were following a path around left field when we found a small garden area with natural grass, scattered purple and white flowers, and butterflies and birds everywhere.

Turning to Armando and Angela, I said, "This is the perfect location for Josh's memorial ceremony. Do you agree?"

Armando and Angela nodded their heads, so from my pocket I pulled a red-colored stone with Josh's name painted in black and handed it to Armando so he could place it in the garden.

During our ceremony, Armando shared beautiful stories about Josh. We learned how much Josh loved children, enjoyed parachuting, and how he aspired to be a child psychologist. Angela shared the impact his preventable death had on their family, and how badly he is missed. Like other parents who lost children needlessly, the pain never ends.

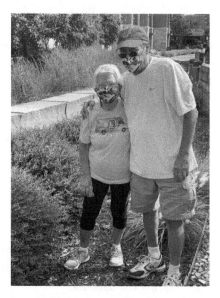

Angela and Armando Nahum
Photo courtesy of Dave Mayer (2020)

Armando shared this passage about his son Josh with me:

Josh was on his final parachuting jump of the day when a cold air density pushed his parachute inward, throwing him to the ground at sixty miles per hour, breaking his femur and fracturing his skull.

This is how our nightmare began.

My wife and I flew to Colorado to be with him. After spending five weeks in ICU and overcoming two cases of MRSA and delirium, Josh seemed to be better and on the road to recovery. His medical team told us we could go home now—that the worst was over. After six days in rehab, Josh developed a high fever and felt nauseous. They sent him back to ICU where they discovered a dangerous gram-negative bacterium present in his cerebral spinal fluid. The last of a series of errors involved the neurosurgeon performing a lumbar puncture prior to a ventriculostomy. Later that night Josh coded. On October 22nd, Josh died, from a series of preventable medical errors.

Over the last fourteen years, Joshua's story has inspired a multitude of health-care workers to just do that "one thing" in the delivery of care: "Change One Thing, Change Everything."

Armando serves on the Presidential Advisory Council for Combating Antibiotic-Resistant Bacteria and the Council for Infection Prevention at the Centers for Disease Control and Prevention (CDC) and continues to educate patients and families about the early warning signs of sepsis. He instructs patients and families who see or experience any signs or symptoms to tell their caregivers, "I suspect sepsis" so a possible diagnosis of sepsis will not be missed, and treatment will not be delayed, as in Josh's case.

After the rock memorial ceremony, we finished our walk and then headed back through The Battery Atlanta shopping area. Still wearing our masks, a young couple in their late thirties crossed the street behind us, not wearing masks. It was easy for me to hear their derogatory comments directed at us about "all the stupid people who believe they need to wear masks." Five months into the pandemic with almost 100,000 Americans already dead from the virus and no end in sight, the political rhetoric and debate about mask wearing was only getting uglier.

The following morning, we were up early and heading south for a nine-hour drive to Tampa Bay and Tropicana Park, home of the Devil Rays. As we drove into the stadium parking lot, I was taken aback by what I saw. The ballpark was a pale-colored concrete bowl shaped stadium, its slanted domed roof reminding me of the spaceships that crashed to earth in the science fiction movie *Independence Day*. Besides the few paintings of Kevin Kiermaier, Blake Snell, Charlie Morton, and Willy Adames in their colorful Tampa Bay uniforms painted on a wall of the ballpark, everything was pale-colored concrete. It was the ugliest ballpark we had visited so far.

Standing in front of the main entrance to Tropicana Park in my Joe Maddon Cubs jersey, my mind drifted back to Maddon's first press conference as the new Cubs manager on November 3rd, 2014. Joe had been the manager of the Tampa Bay Rays from 2006 to 2014 until a contract clause triggered, allowing Maddon to become a manager "free agent." The Chicago Cubs immediately contacted him, convincing Joe to head north and become the sixtieth manager of the Cubs. I and other Cubs fans were eagerly watching that first press conference as Maddon enjoyed the back-and-forth banter with a room full of reporters packed into the Cubby Bear Lounge, a favorite watering hole for Cubs fans located directly across the street from Wrigley Field. When Maddon was asked what excited him about the job, he cited the team's management, the players, and Wrigley Field.

Responding to one reporter's question, Maddon replied "You have to understand something about your ballpark. It is magical."

Maddon continued (and I am paraphrasing Joe): I went to the pitcher's mound to bring in one of our relief pitchers. As I walked back to the dugout, I looked up and was struck by the beauty of a perfect blue sky, the rafters and light stands rising above the ballpark, and all the people sitting in the stands. It was perfect and I slowed my walk to appreciate the moment.

Three local TV reporters met me at the ballpark and interviewed me as I walked around the stadium. My Maddon jersey was now three shades darker than when I first put it on, soaking up the perspiration running down my face and neck. One reporter asked what I thought about "The Trop," the short-ened name used by Rays fans when referring to the ballpark.

"The dome is unique, and I love that it's air conditioned." I replied, trying to not upset any Rays fans watching the interview on TV later that evening.

The reporter laughed before saying, "It's horrible."

"The ultimate purpose of a curriculum in medical education is to address a problem that affects the health of the public."[13]

David E. Kern, Patricia A. Thomas, Donna M. Howard, and Eric B. Bass

Saturday, August 8th, 2020

Total Miles Walked = 1,169
Total Steps = 2,871,626

"In one sentence, will each of the panelists share how we can solve the preventable medical harm crisis."

There it was. The last question from the moderator, posing the million dollar question to each of four panelists at the closing session of an annual Australian Surgical Society meeting, of which I was one of them. I had been invited by Professor Cliff Hughes, a renowned cardiac surgeon and CEO of the Australian New South Wales Clinical Excellence Commission, to be a keynote speaker at the meeting. The theme that year was patient safety, and Cliff had asked me to share our work on disclosure after patient harm and the new four-year patient safety curriculum I had implemented at the University of Illinois's College of Medicine.

Having arrived in Brisbane two days earlier, I was feeling the effects of jet lag from twenty hours of flying to Sydney followed by another two-hour flight

---

[13] David E. Kern, Patricia A. Thomas, Donna M. Howard, and Eric B. Bass, *Curriculum Development for Medical Education: A Six Step Approach* (Baltimore: Johns Hopkins University Press, 1998).

to Brisbane. I was also upset because our hospital's recent CMS Surgical Care Improvement Program (SCIP) outcomes, released the day I boarded a United 747 to Sydney, jumped from 45 percent to over 90 percent for the new quarter. Most leaders would have been elated to see that level of improvement, but I was mad. I served as chair of the SCIP measure committee and expected 100 percent compliance to SCIP measures, which included administering the correct prophylactic antibiotic, administering it within one hour of surgical incision, stopping antibiotics after twenty-four hours, and appropriate hair removal to prevent infection. For the past two years, I had educated, innovated, and pleaded with colleagues about the need to improve our quarterly compliance rates, but all I heard were lame excuses such as "I'm sorry," "We forgot," and "We will do better next time." We were not prioritizing the safety of our patients as we needed to. In 2009, CMS leaders must have been equally frustrated, announcing a financial penalty plan for hospitals with poor SCIP rates. Bingo! The fear of losing revenue spread through the surgeon's lounge like wildfire, everyone now prioritizing the SCIP measures. This CMS financial regulation had been the impetus for change, and our SCIP rates improved dramatically in three short months.

The handheld microphone was still warm in my hand when the moderator finished asking his question. Tired and frustrated, I responded without thinking, the words flowing from my mouth as if a ventriloquist was controlling my thoughts and lips.

"Educate the young and regulate the old!" There it was; my one sentence response, sure to solve the world's patient safety crisis. Realizing what I'd just blurted out, I panicked when glancing down the table to see the stunned looks on my fellow panelists. It was obvious that whatever answer they were formulating in their minds would not top my "in your face" statement. Half the audience laughed; the other half hissed. In that moment, I doubted that I would ever be invited back to Australia.

I still strongly believe that the first part of my response, "Educate the young," is correct. Aviation safety experts David Musson and Robert Helmreich placed a similar emphasis on educating the young in a 2004 article discussing the healthcare quality and safety crisis. The authors recommended healthcare provide education in important risk-reduction domains. "Human factors awareness and interprofessional teamwork training needs to be introduced early in healthcare training—specifically at the medical student and nursing student level as this is the period of acculturation into these professions. Medical and nursing schools must invest in curriculum development to address these issues at the earliest stages of clinical training."[14]

Moments like the one in Australia have defined my patient safety journey, and I was feeling especially melancholy driving from Tampa Bay to Miami. The pandemic had forced us to cancel three weeks of patient safety summer camps that were scheduled to begin that week in Breckinridge, Colorado. I had founded the summer camps in 2010 so that medical students, nursing students, and resident physicians could learn and acquire skills to improve the safety and quality within our healthcare workplace. Time spent with these future healthcare leaders had become my favorite weeks of the year.

Now known as the Academy for Emerging Leaders in Patient Safety (AELPS), the four-day, full-immersion workshops we offer provide residents and students the opportunity to experience hands-on education and training from internationally renowned patient safety and patient advocate leaders on concepts including open and honest communication after unexpected harm, transparency, leadership and mindfulness, patient and family partnerships, just culture, emotional first aid to colleagues, diagnostic error and improvement, interdisciplinary teamwork and communication, system error and human factors engineering, high reliability principles and implementation strategies, quality improvement tools and techniques, informed consent and shared decision making, and the value of stories and narratives to connect the heart and the head of healthcare professionals.

Many of our young scholars in attendance had shared their frustrations over the years, often asking: "Why aren't we learning this important material during our residency?" It was this same frustration coupled with the personal experience of having been young and afraid of harming a patient in a challenging shame and blame culture that had driven me to shape the AELPS program. These important safety and quality competencies and skills were not being taught in their health systems or academic medical settings. Attendees also echoed the feeling of being alone in their pursuit of prioritizing patient safety, their instructors and peers uninterested in learning about the topic because the material was not tested on board exams. Some learners have even

---

[14] David Musson and Robert Helmreich, "Team Training and Resource Management in Health Care: Current Issues and Future Directions," *Harvard Health Policy Review* 5, no. 1 (Spring 2004): 25.

enrolled in our patient safety camps as a last ditch effort to save their career, the abusive nature of our medical culture being too challenging to mental and physical well-being. I have stayed close with many of those who arrived broken to our summer camps, and several have told me that their AELPS week reignited their passion to be a caregiver by reminding them why they chose medicine in the first place. Our AELPS Alumni leave knowing now they are not alone, and that fact, along with our global network of patient safety leaders, is something they take with them for the rest of their careers. This community, a "patient safety family," is available and can be contacted when the toxic medical culture rises up and challenges their spirit to be a healer.

Two recent notes I received from alumni particularly touched my heart, reinforcing the importance of our AELPS work:

"I have to say these last few days at our patient safety summer camp have been eye-opening, and dare I say, life changing. These talks, stories, and reflections have all made me take a step back and realize what it is all about: our patients. It makes me really sad that I have completely lost sight of that in the very little time I have been in residency training. There is no excuse. I could blame exhaustion, long hours, seeing too many patients in too little time, but at the end of the day, there is no excuse for not putting our patients as our number one priority."

And the second one:

"Yesterday was Father's Day. Rolling out of bed, I brewed a much-needed cup of coffee and looked out my window to the inspiring landscape of endless white-capped mountains. This marks the ninth Father's Day that I have spent without my dad, but the mountains and my purpose this week made me feel as though he were standing there with me, sharing our cup of morning coffee, just as we used to.

"I know that despite the growing number of "apology laws," few physicians actually do apologize. This results in families feeling like the events were their fault. I can say from experience that this is a burden that you carry with you for years to come.

"As I got back to my room and put down my books, I mulled over this conversation in my mind. The death of my father has given me the fuel to pursue medicine and patient safety as my career. It has instilled in me passion, energy, and determination. Yet the one thing I have not found in nine years since my father's death is forgiveness. Although I do not hold any one doctor or nurse responsible for the detrimental outcome in my father's care, I have not been able to forgive the team for what happened. I have not been able to go back to the hospital. And as I sat on my bed in the mountains, I realized that I also harbored another feeling: fear. Fear of becoming a physician who does not practice mindfulness, who does not partner with my patients, who does not apologize for my mistakes. I am afraid that, despite my best intentions, I will only continue the vicious cycle. A fear that I will allow my patients to feel as though they are "on an island."

"I put away my computer, got into bed, and took in the gravity of the day. I am so grateful to be here at AELPS among students and faculty who share my passion for patient safety. I could not imagine a more perfect way to spend Father's Day."

I cry every time I read the last reflection.

Other attendees reinforce the reasons why I founded AELPS, sharing testimonials on what the week-long training meant to their professional careers:

(1) "Less than a week after completion of the workshop, I am amazed how I have begun to look at situations in a new light. As I see a safety issue that has occurred, I am able to look past who did it, but rather dig deeper into better understanding the system and how the system failed."

(2) "I was frankly burned out on conferences when I attended the Academy for Emerging Leaders in Patient Safety, and I emerged re-energized to make my hospital safer and to take better care of my patients."

(3) "This workshop was invaluable. In addition to reducing medical errors, it helped me realize that we also need to provide emotional support to our colleagues and team. I have been able to bring back the leadership skills and knowledge I learned to help promote resident wellness and teamwork."

Kim Oates, a patient safety champion and pediatrician, Faculty of Medicine and Health at Sydney Medical School in Australia as well as an AELPS faculty member, recently published a paper that followed up with our Sydney AELPS cohort on the long-term impact attending AELPS had on their careers. Of the 116 scholars who attended in Sydney, 56 percent responded to a survey evaluating their experience on areas of focus like how our curriculum helped them obtain their current position, execute patient safety projects, breakdown hierarchies, and better understand and work side-by-side their patients. Sixty-seven percent agreed AELPS helped them in choosing their career, and 57 percent agreed it had helped them obtain their current position. Overall, Oates and colleagues concluded that "a short, intensive, interdisciplinary program that includes interaction with patient advocates can provide future health leaders with tools to improve communication, understand the patient view, work respectfully with other disciplines and speak up on behalf of the patient."[15] Oates has commented that leadership has never been more important in healthcare, and that there is a growing need to develop future healthcare leaders, especially patient safety experts as the new clinical leader.

With continued support from MedStar Health, The Doctors Company Foundation, The COPIC Foundation, Judith Nowak, Sorrel King, and the Gordon and Betty Moore Foundation, AELPS has continued to grow since its inception. Our Patient Safety Summer Camps have spread internationally as well, and continue to be offered in Sydney, Australia, and Doha, Qatar. AELPS alumni, numbering over 1,400, have formed a growing community of international leaders in patient safety and advocacy, serving as role models for the next generation of healthcare leaders. On a personal note, it is the passion of these young scholars to face the challenges that still prevent open, honest communication and a culture of safety, for example, that recharges my heart and soul each year. Many of our faculty echo similar sentiment. These young people are a diverse, gifted, activated group that reflects a positive version of what healthcare of the future may look like. They give me hope the next generation of healthcare leaders will prioritize patient safety and quality care for patients, while at the same time embracing important efforts like physician and nursing wellness to build a thriving healthcare workforce.

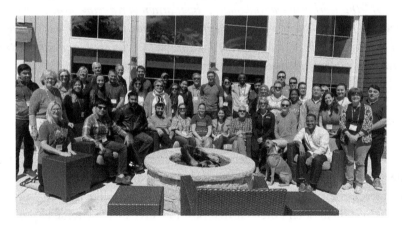

---

[15] Kim Oates, Annette Burgess, and Tyler Clark, "An Interdisciplinary Program for Emerging Leaders in Patient Safety." *The Clinical Teacher* (2022): 1–10. https://doi.org/10.1111/tct.13507

I was disappointed AELPS was not being held in Colorado this week, as it had been the previous eleven years. I was also nervous about this leg of our trip, with southeast Florida having the highest infection rates in the country, adding additional safety concerns for my walk in Miami.

I continued following "Lost on the Frontlines," a web-based, updated collection of healthcare workers who had died from COVID-19 run by *Kaiser Health News* and *The Guardian*. The data from these early deaths indicated "the median age of death from COVID-19 for medical staff was fifty-seven, compared with seventy-eight in the general population. About one-third of the deaths involved concerns over inadequate protective equipment shortages." Healthcare workers were also "at least three times more likely to become infected than the general population."[16]

One of the stories that particularly caught my attention was that of Adeline Fagan:

Adeline Fagan, a twenty-eight-year-old obstetric and gynecologic physician, tested positive for COVID-19 in early July and died in September. She had been working in a Houston emergency department in July, and "a family member said she reused personal protective equipment day after day due to shortages." Dr. Fagan's story is among the other deceased healthcare workers stories included in Lost on the Frontline. About a dozen deaths in their database were physicians under thirty years of age.

In her story, friends mentioned Fagan's comic side: "She was voted by her colleagues 'most likely to be found skipping and singing down the hall to a delivery' and prone to rolling out hammy Scottish and English accents." Fagan "loved delivering babies, loved being part of the happy moment when a baby comes into the world, loved working with mothers." Such a tragic loss—we must never forget them.[17]

Concerns for healthcare worker safety and well-being have escalated since the start of the pandemic. The media continues to share the stress, fatigue, fear, and burnout workers on the front line of care have experienced. Thousands of healthcare workers—nurses, physicians, environmental services personal, and

---

[16] "Lost on the Frontline". KHN.org. Kaiser Health News and The Guardian. August 10,2020.

[17] "Lost on the Frontline". KHN.org. Kaiser Health News and The Guardian. August 10,2020.

emergency medical personnel—lost their lives because of COVID-19. Many more became infected, requiring hospitalization and intensive care admission from the virus. Some public health experts believe the majority of these deaths and hospitalizations would have been preventable if adequate protective equipment (gowns, gloves, and masks), diagnostic tests, and training had been in place at the start of the pandemic.

Wanting to honor Florida healthcare workers who were in the middle of this viral hurricane hitting southeast Florida, I chose to start the day's walk to LoanDepot Park at Mercy Hospital in Coral Gables, Florida. I was excited that my daughter, Carlie, and her fiancé, Brian, walked with me to LoanDepot Park.

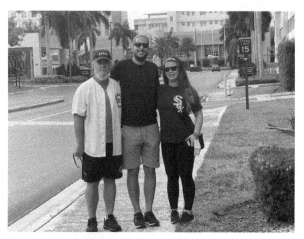

The author with Brian and Carlie
Photo courtesy of Dave Mayer (2020)

After a forty-five-minute drive from Fort Lauderdale to Mercy Hospital, Carlie, Brian, and I started walking northeast on South Miami Avenue while Cathy drove our car to Bay Front Park and walked back to meet us. The smell of palm and citrus fruit trees lining the street infused an uplifting spa-like aroma. Ten-foot-tall yellow and red hibiscus bushes, well-nourished from the Florida humidity, covered half the sidewalk. Hundreds of University of Miami students were out walking, jogging, and biking, the majority not wearing masks and forcing us to walk in the street to avoid contact.

Crossing Biscayne Bay Boulevard, we entered downtown Miami. High-rise condominiums adorned with marble facades and fountains lined both sides of the street, owned by wealthy retirees. All the retirees enjoying their morning walk understood their higher-risk category and wore masks, staying distanced from others passing by.

The downtown Miami landscape changed again. Uber-priced hotels, in towering glass and steel buildings, shaded us from the sun rising to the east. High-end steak and seafood restaurants mixed with designer boutique shops occupied every available parcel of real estate along Brickell Avenue. The absence of large cruise ships in the Port of Miami was another reminder of COVID's impact on our lives. Prior to the pandemic, tens of thousands of cruise-goers would be embarking and disembarking from fifteen to twenty ships lined up on any given Saturday. This morning, the port was empty, the pandemic forcing major cruise lines to shut down.

Around four miles in, we arrived at Bayfront Park, a large community park on the Biscayne Bay waterfront. Park benches shaded by mature palm trees were abundant throughout the thirty-two-acre property, and the cool, salty breeze off the water made the park a cooling spot during humid summer days.

My walk across the country continued to reinforce the beauty, kindness, and resilience of many people I met along the way. These qualities were demonstrated again at Bayfront Park. Approaching the entrance to a public bathroom, the smell of fresh bleach almost knocked me over, making my eyes water. Once inside, one would have thought the restroom was located in one of the high-end hotels we passed earlier—the steel sinks, mirrors, and shower facilities shiny and spotless. Exiting the bathroom, a middle-aged environmental service worker handed me a small bottle of hand sanitizer. The city of Miami was giving hand-sanitizer bottles to everyone who used the park's facilities, something I had not seen in other cities.

Rewashing my hands with the sanitizer, I thanked the man. "What a great idea! Does the city provide you enough bottles to give out to everyone?"

"They do. I haven't run out yet." The worker replied through his mask. "Many homeless people live in the park and use the bathroom facilities. They have an elevated risk of getting COVID."

"I have to tell you, this is the cleanest public bathroom I have ever been in." I thanked him for his effort.

Even with his mask on, I could tell he had a big smile on his face. "Thank you, senor. I am in there every ten minutes wiping everything down with the bleach packs they give us. Another way to keep the virus from spreading."

"Stay safe too," I told him, and left him to his work. The excitement and pride he exuded trying to keep people safe from the virus that was ravaging south Florida was the highlight of my walk in Miami.

Leaving Bayfront Park, the neighborhood changed again. Gone were the expensive high-rise condominiums, the five-star hotels and mega-yachts, now replaced by boarded-up storefronts and sidewalks covered with broken glass. We were entering the neighborhood known as Little Havana, one of the poorest areas in Miami. Every building we now passed was covered with spray-painted graffiti and gang logos. Hundreds of homeless Hispanic and Cuban people lined the streets, many sitting on curbs littered with cans and bottles. Few wore masks or social distanced from one another, making me wonder how many from this community had already died from COVID. With south Florida experiencing the nation's highest COVID infection rates, this segment of my walk brought those concerns to life, worried I was walking through a petri dish of pandemic infection.

After walking two more miles, the roof of LoanDepot Park appeared off to the west. The streets surrounding the stadium were blocked, COVID testing being done in parking lots outside the ballpark. Three local TV station reporters were waiting to interview us, each taking turns firing off questions about my walk. The camera crews filmed our rock memorial service remembering a radiology tech from Jackson Memorial Hospital in Miami who died of COVID-19, honoring Holy Cross Hospital where Carlie and Brian were treated for COVID-19, and all first responders who continued to put their lives on the line every day. Painted rocks for each were placed in a small garden outside the main entrance gate, Carlie sharing thoughts about each.

I had now walked to fifteen of the thirty Major League ballparks. Over five months, I completed forty television, radio, and newspaper interviews on patient safety and preventable medical deaths, sharing stories about those lost. My plan was working even though the callouses on my feet and the pain in my lower back were reaching heightened levels of discomfort.

"They may forget your name, but they will never
forget how you made them feel."

Maya Angelou

Thursday, August 20th, 2020

Miles walked = 1,232
Steps = 3,002,738

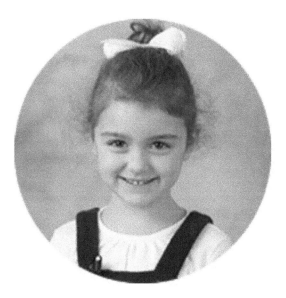

Gabby Galbo
Photo courtesy of Tony and Liz Galbo

It was dawn when Cathy and I packed up the car and began our drive from the Sunshine State to Cincinnati, home of the Reds. As we neared the state line, our conversation turned to Cincinnati, where we planned to hold a memorial service in honor of Gabby Galbo, whose death at the age of five was attributed to medical error, misdiagnosis, and miscommunication. After leaving Cincinnati, we were meeting her parents, Liz and Tony, in Monticello, Illinois, for a dedication ceremony.

Cathy and I have three children and four grandchildren. To think about the gravity of this kind of loss is not only uncomfortable—it's unthinkable and unbearable. Gabby, who died in 2012, would have been graduating from eighth grade and preparing to start high school in the fall. I try to imagine her parents, Liz and Tony Galbo, dealing with the devasting loss of a child, but I quickly realize it isn't something most people understand unless they've been there. They must miss Gabby's beautiful smile, her brown hair pulled back in a ponytail with a bow holding it in place, her tiny voice that liked to sing, and the sound of her giggling when she thought something was funny. Cathy pulls up a photo of her on her phone when we stop for the night and I wonder if Gabby's friends and family still picture her being five, or if they see her as a teenager and imagine what she might be like today, her style of dress, her favorite movie, song, or dreams for the future. It's like someone you adore suddenly leaves and their "goneness" is so huge you keep tripping on it.

The pandemic showed no signs of easing. New forecasts called for a third and larger COVID spike in the fall. We'd been on the road for fifty-six consecutive days and while racking up Bonvoy Marriott points, we missed our king bed, our feather pillows, and our bathroom. The hotel bedsheets, blankets, and pillowcases having an industrial hotel smell and the bathrooms with small bars of soap in plastic wrapping were wearing on us. We were tired of living out of suitcases, wondering what clothes we had previously worn, and eating at fast-food restaurants, missing a home-cooked meal and not wearing masks between bites. But, we had more cities and stadiums to visit, more families to walk with, remembering those lost.

After checking into a downtown Cincinnati hotel, we changed and headed out for a six-mile afternoon walk. It had been over twenty years since my last trip to Cincinnati, when I gave a talk at Cincinnati Children's Hospital. Cathy and I had the downtown area to ourselves, the pandemic continuing to keep people working from home. As we walked, I was enthralled by the beauty of the city. Unlike most big cities, with their expansive downtown streets concentrated with clusters of skyscrapers and a plethora of restaurants and bars, the smaller Cincinnati downtown area was easy to navigate. Its tree-lined riverfront parks, museums, and bike paths give the city a neighborly feel.

The next morning, dressed in my retro '70s Reds jersey, we walked from downtown Cincinnati to Paul Brown Stadium, home of the Cincinnati Bengals football team, looping back along the riverfront. The park benches were occupied by early morning book readers enjoying a cup of coffee. Others sat on blankets, sharing breakfast from open picnic baskets. Cyclists crowded the bike paths, the serious on high-priced titanium bikes in full biking regalia, others enjoying a casual ride through the city. The riverfront was providing a few hours of normalcy for residents despite the pandemic. As we neared Great America Ballpark, the home of the Cincinnati Reds baseball team, I was struck by the stadium's majestic look, the ballpark appearing to dwarf other ballparks we had visited. Sitting along the Ohio River, the stadium's three levels of decks span from the left field foul pole to the right field foul pole, matching the height of downtown office buildings built behind it.

The ballpark brought back many great memories of "The Big Red Machine," the nickname given to one of the greatest baseball teams to ever play the game. The Reds won six division titles, four National League pennants, and two World Series in the '70s. The large bronze action statutes featuring Hall of Fame players reminded me of ballplayers I grew up cheering for. Johnny Bench, the fourteen-time all-star catcher, twice winning the Most Valuable Player award. Joe Morgan, considered one of the best second baseman to ever play the game. Pete Rose, known as "Charlie Hustle," the all-time MLB leader in hits with 4,256. Four TV reporters met us at the main gate, wanting to interview me about my walk. All four stations followed me down the right field side of the ballpark where I found a garden, the lawn perfectly manicured with colorful flowers circling the perimeter. Pulling a yellow painted memorial rock from my pocket with the name Gabby written on it, I shared the tragic loss of five-year-old Gabby Galbo to medical harm with the four reporters before laying the stone on the grass.

After leaving Cincinnati, we arrived at Nicks Park in Monticello, Illinois, where Liz and Tony Galbo were waiting for us. The park is home to Gabby's Gazebo. Built in 2017, the white balustraded gazebo is decorated with colorful metal butterflies on the sides and roof. The gazebo is dedicated to their daughter, Gabby, who loved butterflies, especially monarchs. Gabby died at five years of age from sepsis because of Rocky Mountain spotted fever that went undiagnosed at a hospital. The sidewalk leading up to the structure has Gabby's footprints pressed into the cement, as if she were here with us. We held a memorial service for Gabby, under the doomed roof with a moment of silence before leaving a painted rock in the flower garden.

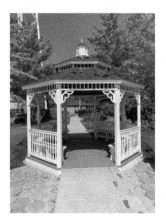 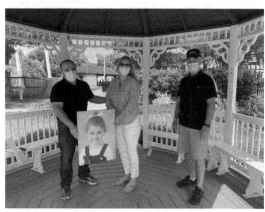

Gabby's Gazebo; Tony and Liz Galbo with the author
Photo courtesy of Dave Mayer (2020)

Tony shared this story about their daughter Gabby:

On May 11th, 2012, at 5:00pm
    Here I am—sitting in the passenger seat of the funeral director's vehicle, escorting my daughter's body home. At this very moment we should have been aboard a plane on our way to Orlando, Florida, for Gabby's first cruise adventure—a vacation she persuaded all of us to take.
    Eleven days ago, Gabby was a healthy, vivacious five-year-old little girl counting down the days for our cruise. I sit here now, at her funeral, trying to figure out what went wrong and how my daughter died. How did eight doctors and six nurses fail? Over the course of a week, a pediatrician had seen her twice, four ER doctors examined her, along with four pediatric intensivists. How did she slip through the cracks and safety nets that were supposed to catch mistakes? There were multiple visits to healthcare providers before Gabby was admitted to the hospital. Misdiagnoses and a series of other errors led to medical harm; labs drawn, but never read, being discharged with abnormal labs, a dangerous differential diagnosis not treated, and not initiating a transfer to a children's hospital until the

family demanded it. We were pacified or dismissed. We had always been a family that received second, even third opinions, but when your child is sick, and medical professionals keep assuring you not to worry, you go against your gut feeling that something is wrong. What if they had shared vital information with us about her differential diagnosis, read her labs correctly, discussed them with us, and been transparent about their many mistakes?

We'd still have our beautiful Gabby.

Preventable medical harm happens. It begins with the smallest error and snowballs into an irreversible catastrophic nightmare. When your loved one dies from medical harm, it cripples your family, destroys your foundation, and your trust for the medical establishment. I wake up every day feeling guilty that I'm alive and Gabby is gone.

Gabby, we love and miss you so much....

Love, Dad and Mom

Since the tragic loss of their daughter Gabby, the Galbos have dedicated their lives to making care safer for others through their legislative work with congressional leaders focused on early sepsis detection and timely treatment. Sepsis claims about 300,000 lives and costs about $41.5 billion to fight in the United States. Despite their gut-wrenching loss, they continue to fight every day to reduce preventable medical harm and make care safer for others.

Sunday, August 23rd, 2020

I was joined by nationally recognized patient safety leaders for my nine-mile walk from Guaranteed Rate Field, home to the Chicago White Sox, to Wrigley Field, home of my beloved Cubs. Dr. Tim McDonald, a longtime friend and colleague, joined me again today. Tim is one of the leading global providers of intelligent patient safety solutions, whose research focuses on the principled approach to patient harm and the normalization of compassionate honesty. He greeted me wearing his Mark Buehrle #56 Sox jersey to complement my Ryne Sandberg #22 Cubby shirt—the crosstown classic—the Windy City Showdown.

Our group started walking north on South Shields Avenue heading toward downtown Chicago. Our route took us through Chinatown with its brightly painted restaurants and shops, walking under the red and gold "Welcome to

Chinatown" sign spanning South Wentworth Avenue. Shade from the financial district skyscrapers in the South Loop provided welcome relief from a cloudless sky before exiting downtown and continuing up North Clark Street.

About a mile from Wrigley Field, we were joined by Brad Schwartz. Brad is a medical malpractice attorney who, in 2004, lost portions of all four of his limbs because of delayed sepsis diagnosis and medical error. After six months in the hospital and a year in physical rehabilitation learning to use prosthetic legs and arms, he founded Greater National Advocates, becoming a national leader working to eliminate preventable medical harm. Brad walked with us the last mile, making our walk today even more special.

Brad shared the following passage with me:

When I heard Dave was walking across the country for patient safety and stopping at ballparks along the way, some obvious metaphors came to mind. Baseball, like medicine, is a team sport that requires every player to be focused and game-day ready. Teammates rely on each other and a weak spot in the lineup can easily be exploited. Education, training, and experience only go so far as the best teams have players who are not only highly skilled, but in sync with each other.

Like athletic ability in baseball, clinical skills in the healthcare environment mean nothing unless care is coordinated. Success requires not only years of training, but also ongoing communication and attention to detail. That's why baseball players are not left to fend for themselves on the field. There is a manager and there are coaches who watch every move with a careful analytic eye. And, if something goes slightly awry, the team takes a break and talks it over on the mound to make sure everyone has their eye on the ball.

In 2004, I became the victim of a cascade of errors in an emergency room. In short, I received no attention for almost 10 hours while I went into septic shock. It was the lack of oversight ... the absence of a second set of eyes and ears that caused the systemic breakdown that almost took my life. My emergency room ordeal left me a quadruple amputee, and it became my life mission to prevent these types of errors from happening to anyone else.

I'm the president and founder of Greater National Advocates, a nonprofit foundation that promotes independent patient advocacy and connects patients and families with healthcare support. The goal is to provide patients and loved ones with access to experienced advocates who can help manage care and minimize risk, just like the coaches and managers in baseball. When it comes to preventing medical errors, I believe independent patient advocates can make a significant impact. They are there to make sure every member of the healthcare team is on their game, so that nobody drops the ball. And if they do drop it, advocates make sure somebody is there to pick it up and make a play before the game becomes unwinnable.

On behalf of patients, families, and survivors of medical error, I applaud the efforts of Dave Mayer for not only talking the talk, but actually walking the walk to bring attention to the dire need for safe medical care. I invite all readers to learn about independent patient advocacy at GNANOW.ORG and help spread the work about this important emerging profession.

As we approached Wrigley Field and the corner of Clark and Addison, I could see three television cameras mounted on tripods and a microphone stand six feet in front of the cameras. I asked Brad to share with the reporters why he was walking with us today. Like others who have suffered preventable medical harm, Brad did a better job of relaying the importance of patient safety and preventable harm than I could ever have done.

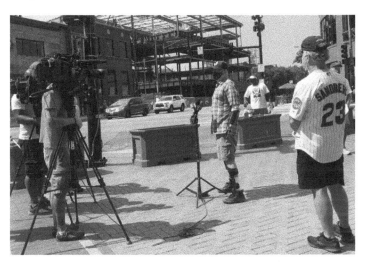

Brad Schwartz
Photo courtesy of Dave Mayer (August 2020)

"First, do no harm" ("Primum non nocere")

Origin uncertain

Tuesday, September 15th, 2020

Miles walked = 1,414
Total Steps = 3,371,606

We left Chicago on August 23rd on our way back to Arizona, stopping in Omaha, Nebraska, with a five-mile walk to TD Ameritrade Park, home of the annual College World Series tournament, and then Denver, Colorado, where we walked nine miles, finishing at Coors Field. By the time we arrived in Phoenix, our sixty-eight-day trip totaled 13,328 miles, which included visits to twenty-five states, sixteen Major League stadiums, ten Cactus League parks, two Grapefruit League ballparks, three minor league parks, and a handful of college and professional football stadiums.

I remember the first night back, being excited to sleep in our own king-size bed. We no longer kept our clothes in open suitcases, sorting them each night for our next walk, searching for that specific shirt or shorts we wanted to wear or for a clean pair of socks, underwear, or walking shoes. We arranged them in piles, always trying to locate a certain item we were missing—digging our way through them like a dog who is looking for a buried bone. Locating hotels along our route with laundry facilities became more important than knowing how many miles it was to the next gas station. We had a couple weeks to unwind before the next leg of the trip—flying to Washington DC on September 17th for the World Health Organization's (WHO) World Patient Safety Day. Established in 2019, patients, families, caregivers, healthcare leaders, and policy makers come together on September 17th to raise awareness about patient safety around the world. Monuments and buildings are lit up in orange, showing unity to a goal of zero preventable harm.

COVID infection and death rates soared, and predictions for the coming spike terrified most people. I was nervous thinking about flying back to Washington DC, remembering my daughter Carlie and her fiancé, Brian, both young and healthy, who were still suffering long-term respiratory complications six months after being infected. I had read hundreds of gut-wrenching stories about those lost to the virus, doing everything possible to stay safe. Southwest Airlines continued to keep middle seats open but even with masks and shields, and hand sanitizers, the thought of being in an enclosed metal tube containing about one hundred people for five hours didn't seem safe. Despite federal mandatory mask requirements, there were always some dissenters who chose to ignore the mandates by wearing their masks around their necks or taking four hours to finish drinking their cups of coffee and others abandoning their face masks, hoping no one would notice or care.

My DC plan involved walking seven-to-ten miles each day followed by shorter afternoon walks with friends and patient safety leaders from all over the country. The first morning included a brisk walk along the grassy DC Mall and reflection pond, visiting war memorials, and honoring veterans. According to the Department of Veterans Affairs, over 20,000 military veterans died from COVID-19 in VA Hospitals or in hospitals connected to the VA health system across the country.[18]

Arriving at a long black granite wall, I studied the long list of names of those who lost their lives during the Vietnam War. Over 58,000 names of U.S. soldiers are remembered at the Vietnam Memorial. Many other brave soldiers whose names are not included on the wall suffered long-term physical and psychological harm. We cannot forget their sacrifice.

Walking farther down the mall, the life-size statues of military personnel in uniform, covered by rain ponchos, walking through bushes and tall green grass, rifles in one hand and walkie talkies in the other, stopped me in my tracks. The scene, part of the Korean War Veterans Memorial, highlights the challenges and sacrifices made by those who served. The soldiers appeared so life-like, I envisioned myself in a Korean jungle watching the procession.

---

[18] Shane III, Leo. VA tops 20,000 COVID deaths in less than two years. www.militarytimes. com. February 15th, 2021.

Reading the words on the wall next to the statues, "Freedom Is Not Free," the realization that hundreds of thousands have died protecting our freedom over the last century is sobering and at times unrecognized and unappreciated.

On Wednesday afternoon, twenty masked patient safety advocates began walking down Freedom Plaza to the Capitol Building. Few people were out on the streets as we headed down Pennsylvania Avenue, distancing ourselves eight feet apart, holding on to a two-hundred-foot orange rope. We looked like a giant tangerine centipede, holding our Patient Safety Movement Foundation banner at the front of the line, the remaining eighteen advocates holding Unite for Safe Care posters with their free hands.

Groups of twenty-five or more were not allowed to congregate on DC streets because of the pandemic, so we limited our group to twenty. A cameraman ran along the street next to us, filming and throwing out questions about patient safety and our mission, trying to learn more about why we were here and what we hoped to accomplish. Tony Galbo shared the story of his daughter Gabby, Carole Hemmelgarn spoke about her daughter Alyssa, Vonda Vaden-Bates reminisced about her late husband, Yogiraj, and I spoke about the need for a safe healthcare system for both patients and healthcare workers.

The next day our team was granted a permit to plant 2,000 orange flags on the Capitol Building lawn. Each flag had the Unite for Safe Care logo on one side and the name of someone lost to preventable medical harm on the other. We planted our flags on the Capitol Building lawn, signifying the more than 250,000 people lost every year because of preventable harm. I stepped back to view our orange garden. The landscape of the flags against the Capitol Building backdrop triggered similar emotions I experienced at the Vietnam and Korean Memorials. The flags were our memorial to the hundreds of thousands lost each year to preventable harm. Congressional leaders in the building behind our memorial have the ability to make care safer. Patients and caregivers need them to act now.

One of those 2,000 orange flags had the name Noah Lord written on it. Noah had his tonsils removed at four years of age. After the tonsillectomy, he was discharged home but continued to cough and refused to drink or eat over the following three days. His mother Tanya took Noah back to the emergency department but was reassured all was well. Four hours after returning home, while lying on the couch he lifted his head and called "Mommy!" before coughing and bleeding profusely from his mouth and nose. The bleeding was so severe, blood clots began obstructing his airway. EMT was called but Noah died before they arrived.

Tanya Lord is a national patient safety advocate and good friend who shared this story about Noah.

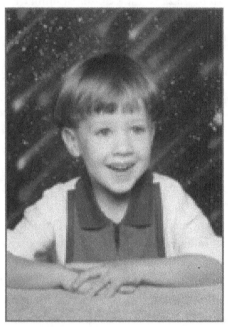

Noah Lord
Photo courtesy of Tanya Lord

"First do no harm" I heard this phrase for the first time after my son, Noah, died at four years old from a series of medical errors following a tonsillectomy. My grief, anguish and anger only seemed to build. I kept asking myself, "How did this happen?"

Noah was a gentle, loving spirit. There was no teaching him "stranger danger" because he never met a stranger, young or old—they were all his friends.

It wasn't long before I realized that the enormous amount of negative emotion and energy I carried wasn't serving a purpose in my life and didn't reflect who Noah was or the kind of legacy my son would approve of. So, I dealt with the anger, learned how to manage my grief by allowing my anguish and pain to honor his short life. As I completed my master's and then my PhD, I began to understand how medical errors happen and how we can learn from them. Healthcare providers need to engage patients and families in their clinical work. Zero harm comes from following the oath.

Harm is done by a human working in a faulty system.

Harm is done every time a mom says, "Something is wrong," and she is not heard.

Harm is done when tears of a patient are met with frustration or are ignored.

Harm is done when a lonely, scared patient is left in silence.

Harm is done when a patient is clinically treated but not known.

Harm is done because healthcare has forgotten to include love in everything they do. It is the clinicians and staff who love their patients openly who do the least harm. When love is primary, mistakes are lessened, forgiven, and healed. Noah showed love to everyone. As an infant, he raised his arms to strangers and giggled when they picked him up. It is OK to be Noah and demonstrate love to patients by listening and showing someone they are important, and what they think and feel is important. Loving patients may seem like a huge risk, but it is in love that we improve safety. Let this be Noah's legacy.

Tanya shares that improvements in patient safety can be achieved "by engaging patients and families" as partners on the care team. Some in healthcare do not welcome patient and family participation into our safety efforts and when we do not welcome their participation, four-year-old children like Noah die.

Saturday, September 19th, 2020

I arrived Saturday morning in Philadelphia, a two-hour drive from DC, to begin my eight-mile roundtrip walk from Freedom Plaza and the Liberty Bell in downtown Philly to Citizens Bank Park, home of the Phillies.

My Cubs jersey no longer kept me warm without a jacket. The mild temperatures, along with a stiff frigid wind out of the east, forced me to wear a coat over my Ryne Sandberg jersey. Though invisible to people on the street, my jersey was the perfect choice for today's walk. The all-star and Hall of Fame Cubs second baseman began his playing career in the Phillies organization before being traded to the Cubs. To me, Sandberg was the epitome of a baseball player, working hard on his skills while never complaining or causing problems. Nicknamed "Ryno," Sandberg played fifteen years for the Cubs and was selected to ten consecutive all-star games while winning nine consecutive Golden Glove Awards. In 1990, Sandberg led the league in home runs, a rarity for second basemen, slugging forty round-trippers. Cubs fans never forget the 1984 nationally televised game when, in the bottom of the ninth inning, Sandberg homered off Cardinal ace reliever Bruce Sutter, sending the game into extra innings. The Cards scored two runs in the top of the tenth inning, but in the bottom of the inning Sandberg tied the game by homering off Sutter again and the Cubs went on to win the game in the eleventh inning. After finishing his career with the Cubs, he became manager of the Philadelphia Phillies from 2013 to 2015. Sandberg resigned in his third season as the Phillies struggled with the worst record in the major leagues.

The colder temperatures did not keep the locals indoors. South Philadelphia was alive with basketball and baseball games being played at all the community parks. The streets were crowded with early morning shoppers making rounds at their favorite markets. I passed wooden tables, set up on the sidewalks, with all types of fresh fish, meat, and produce piled on crushed ice. The palpable energy and excitement in the South Philly neighborhood was like caffeine to me, my walking cadence now faster than normal. The scene reminded me of the movie *Rocky* when Rocky Balboa would do similar walks, passing the same sidewalk markets in South Philly where he lived. I began humming the theme song from *Rocky* expecting to hear, "Yo Adrian!" being shouted off in the distance.

When I arrived at Citizens Bank Park, I walked around the ballpark passing the statues of Philly greats like Richie Ashburn, Robin Roberts, Mike Schmidt, and Steve Carlton. Growing up, I was a Richie Ashburn fan. His name was inscribed on the inside pocket of one of my baseball mitts and he played center field, the position I yearned to play with the Chicago Cubs. Ashburn wasn't a player who hit for power but he found a way to get on base, totaling over 2,500 hits in his Hall of Fame career. In addition to those four Philadelphia all-star ballplayers, there is also a fifth statue of Harry Kalas, the legendary Philly radio broadcaster.

Before walking back to downtown Philadelphia, I pulled a baby-blue-painted rock out of my jacket pocket for the memorial service and moment of silence, this morning remembering Lola Jayden Fitch, a newborn child who died from preventable medical harm.

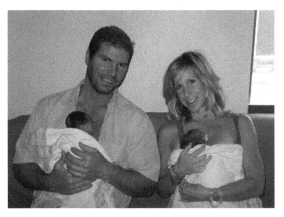

Alan and Cathy Fitch with their twins Lola and Grayson
Photo courtesy of Cathy Motley-Fitch

Cathy Motley-Fitch is a national patient safety leader who teaches health-care workers how to use effective communication skills to reduce harm. She shared the following passage with me:

Our twins, Lola Jayden and her brother Grayson Howard were born at thirty-two weeks. They were early, yet there were no apparent complications. They were admitted to the NICU for observation and called feeders and growers, a term used in the NICU for babies needing more time to grow and mature. We had a beautiful week as we loved, laughed, and sang to them, hardly leaving their sides.

One week later, on June 5th, 2009, our world turned upside down. I stayed home to rest but called the hospital several times to check on the babies. Each time, they reassured me they were doing fine. When I called to say goodnight, the nurse's tone was different. I was told my daughter would be fine but was "feeling kind of 'punk.'" Throughout the night, Lola's health spiraled out of control and within six hours, I found myself holding my daughter as she took her last breath and died. We were left in shock and discovered her death was the result of a series of miscommunications, misdiagnoses, and medical errors—a tragic situation that could have been prevented.

Our daughter, Lola became one of the estimated 210,000 to 400,000 preventable deaths in the United States caused by medical mistakes each year.

We made a choice to partner with the hospital where she died and share her story in efforts to impact change and make care safer for others. That partnership has brought us healing and inspiration.

"An ounce of prevention is worth a pound of cure."

Benjamin Franklin

October 24th, 2020

Miles walked = 1,660
Steps = 3,907,190

My original plan had me continuing to New York and Boston to visit Yankee Stadium, Citi Field, and Fenway Park, but COVID infection rates had skyrocketed in New York City, forcing travel embargoes for those living outside the state. This segment of my walk had special meaning for me, and I was disappointed it wouldn't happen. On a family trip to New York in 1964, my father was able to snag two tickets to the all-star game at Shea Stadium that year, the park now called Citi Field. Sitting in the second deck of the right field bleachers, watching the game's best players—Mickey Mantle, Harmon Killebrew, Willie Mays, Roberto Clemente, and the Cubs own Billy Williams—together on one field created memories I never forgot. My walks to those three ballparks would have to wait.

By the fall of 2020, Houston and Dallas were seeing the most infections from a third COVID spike. My upcoming walk at Minute Maid Park, home of the Astros, and Globe Life Field, home of the Texas Rangers, would also have to be postponed. This resilient virus challenged my goal of walking to all thirty Major League ballparks by mid-February when I envisioned hitting the magic number of 2,452 miles walked—the distance from San Diego, California, to Jacksonville Beach, Florida.

I had walked almost 1,700 miles over 220 straight days, leaving me about 770 miles remaining before arriving in Jacksonville Beach, Florida. My walks in Arizona averaged eight to nine miles a day, approximately three and a half miles per hour, depending on the degree of pain radiating from my hips or back, but I continue to push myself to go that extra mile. I felt a need to pound and pace myself, fighting days when mental exhaustion would take over, making it difficult to just lace up my shoes. I walk scenic routes, a half-abandoned landscape full of dreams, ideas, and adventures, occasionally greeted by a rattlesnake, playing dead hoping to avoid confrontation or coiled and ready to attack, its rattling tail crackling like electrical wires stopping me in my tracks. Coyotes and javelinas frequently cross my path while hawks circle overhead looking for prey. I'm pushing toward Jacksonville Beach, and I need to keep moving, staying in shape, both body and mind—always one step ahead of the virus. I'm determined to complete my walk across America.

The safest option, based on the rising COVID infection and death rates, was to drive to California and hit the four remaining ballparks there. My walk began last February in San Diego and Petco Park, the city bubbling with energy before the pandemic hit, but I still needed to walk to Angel Stadium in Anaheim, Dodger Stadium in Los Angeles, Oracle Park in San Francisco, and the Oakland Coliseum as COVID rates continued to handcuff outdoor city activity. A five-hour drive to Los Angeles, followed by a second five-hour drive north, seemed like an easy feat—much shorter than our last sixty-seven-day driving trip.

Giant dirty thunderheads and the smell of smoke welcomed us to Newport Beach. Orange and red flames rising above the mountains, just east of Irvine, lit up the sky as the black smoke from forest fires blew toward the Pacific Ocean. Eighty to one hundred mile per hour Santa Ana winds on top of the mountains fueled the fires and hampered firefighters from gaining control of the flames. News reports of poor air quality warned people with lung conditions to stay inside, my facemask hopefully providing additional protection from the smoke. I ran my finger through a coat of ash covering a white Toyota parked on the street, leaving a foot-long line on the hood. After each coughing spasm during my morning walks, I wondered how much ash was making it through my mask and being deposited in my lungs with each breath. My walk had already been challenged by a pandemic, racial protests and riots, religious hatred, and political division, and now uncontrolled forest fires. What was next? Locusts? Vermin? Frogs? As the challenges mounted, I thought back to better days, my walks with family and friends elevating my spirits and countering moments of depression.

The forest fires impacting Irvine stayed south of Los Angeles, minimizing our respiratory concerns, so on Tuesday morning, October 27th, Cathy and

I drove from Newport Beach to Los Angeles for our eleven-mile roundtrip walk to Dodgers Stadium.

I walked along Hollywood and Sunset Boulevard before passing through Asian and Hispanic neighborhoods that call east L.A. home. I slowed my pace, browsing a series of street art, an exhibition of brightly colored murals and mosaics displayed on brick walls of single-story buildings. Each passing neighborhood displayed and shared its deep cultural history: religion, community, and family—embracing the importance of life. One exhibit, *The Wall that Talks*, blended symbols from Aztec, Mayan, Native American, and other cultural iconography all in unity with one another. It had a large sign above it that read Arroyo Furniture. My favorite one, a mural tucked away in Boyle Heights, featured a vibrant, cubist-like portrait of Lakers legend Kobe Bryant. The artist used hard angles executed in blues and purples giving the impression of an image existing in both space and time.

My fixation on the mosaics was halted by the distinct call of a crowing rooster. The cock-a-doodle-doo was coming from somewhere behind a four-foot chainlink fence on my left where I spotted a thick eight-foot-tall hedge just behind the fence, keeping Peeping Toms like me from invading the homeowner's privacy. An opening between two bushes allowed me a view of a six-foot-tall wooden chicken coop sitting a few feet from a one-story home. Ten to twenty hens and roosters roamed the property pecking at seeds scattered on the ground. Growing up, my visual recollection of Hollywood and Vine, the famous Sunset Strip, came from television shows like *77 Sunset Strip*, the popular early '60s detective show starring Edd Byrnes (yes with two d's), who played Kookie, and Efrem Zimbalist Jr. The episodes were sprinkled with scenes of the rich and famous shopping and dining at high-end boutiques and restaurants on the strip. Roosters and chickens roaming the streets along Sunset Boulevard never entered my mind.

The city of Los Angeles was abuzz today because the Dodgers were playing in game six in the 2020 World Series. Fans wearing Dodger-blue jerseys and baseball caps lined the streets as we approached the stadium, many shouting "Go Dodgers" and high-fiving each other as they passed. The Dodgers had a 3–2 lead and their die-hard faithful were already planning their post-win celebration activities. City officials and Dodger management were one step ahead of the overzealous fans. At Dodger Stadium, we were greeted by security guards who had blocked all entrances into the parking lots, fearing fans would assemble around the empty park and cause a COVID super-spreader situation. And they did. Wide-eyed Angelinos decked out in blue watched and cheered from a parking lot outside Dodger Stadium as the storied franchise captured its first World Series title since 1988. Crowds—some from their cars, others on lawn chairs—watched, cheered, and celebrated the night, bringing back great memories of 2016 when I celebrated the Cubs' World Series victory with Chicago fans in Cleveland. We attempted to walk around the ballpark, looking for any entrance gate that might allow us closer access to the ballpark, but we never made it past the main parking lot entrance.

Before leaving, despite the tumult all around us, the primary mission of my walk was patient and health worker safety. I pulled from my pocket a yellow painted rock with the name Nile written on it in black ink and placed it on the manicured lawn under the blue and white Dodger Stadium sign. Nile Moss died from a hospital-acquired infection followed by delayed detection and treatment of sepsis, another tragic loss that was caused by preventable medical harm. Nile's parents, Carole and Ty, have dedicated their lives to making care safer for others by raising awareness, early detection, and education about sepsis. Through their work, in 2008 California passed SB1058, called Nile's Law, requiring hospitals to screen, measure, and report hospital infections.

Nile's parents, Carole and Ty, wrote this passage about their son, Nile.

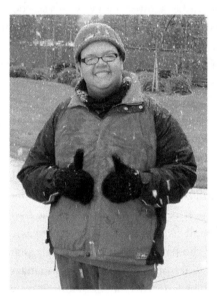

Nile Moss
Photo courtesy of Carole Moss

Nile came into the world needing to depend on the knowledge and benefits of the medical system. He was born with a treatable medical condition, hydrocephalus, an abnormal buildup of fluid in the ventricles (cavities) within the brain. But that wasn't the cause of his death, just a setback in his life that he overcame with love, joy, and sound medical treatment.

As parents we were his advocates from the day he was born, always involved and informed with his medical condition. During his short life of fifteen years, he left a lasting impression on everyone he met. His grateful heart and joyful spirit inspired teachers, doctors, nurses, family, friends, athletes, and the musicians who loved him—Nile's Project band.

Nile had a full, prosperous life; he traveled internationally and lived every day to the fullest. That changed overnight when he contracted a bacterial infection known as MRSA (methicillin-resistant Staphylococcus aureus), from a visit to a children's hospital. Within forty-eight hours of his annual exam, including an MRI, Nile displayed flu-like symptoms that progressed over seventy-two hours. He was admitted to Children's Hospital with a fever of 104°F.

At the time, we were unaware of the existence of an MRSA epidemic, which plagued hospitals across the nation. It wasn't long before the infection progressed to full-blown sepsis resulting in organ failure. If we had known then what we now know about MRSA and sepsis, our son might still be with us.

Nile taught everyone the power of faith and hope. He inspired us to advocate for patient safety within the medical system and beyond. We have dedicated our lives to creating safer hospitals across the country, raising sepsis awareness, including early detection, and education about effective treatment programs. In 2008, California passed SB1058, called Nile's Law, requiring hospitals to screen, measure, and report infections.

We use the language of music to tell our story. Nile's life and music inspired our first album and public awareness concerts. "Keep a smile in your heart, we're gonna do great things."

Driving back to Orange County after remembering Nile, orange skies and ash-dusted neighborhoods continued to plague my walk across America. Our walk to Angels Stadium was originally scheduled for Thursday, but the smoke from nearby fires created a health hazard for anyone venturing outside. On Friday, firefighters gained control of most of the wildfires and promised worried residents an improvement in air quality by the weekend.

Feeling safer, we headed out Saturday morning, starting our walk at Chapman University, the academic home of President and Dean Ronald Jordan, who leads the pharmacy safety programs that target three of the most common causes of medication errors: (1) dispensing incorrect medications, dosages, or forms; (2) miscalculating dosages; and (3) missed drug interactions or contraindications. Our route included a walk to Children's Hospital of Orange County (CHOC), then off to University of California Irvine (UCI) Medical Center, before finishing the seven-mile leg at Angel Stadium in Anaheim.

I was excited to have Joe Kiani, the founder and former CEO of the Patient Safety Movement Foundation (PSMF), walking with me this morning. Joe's vision of, and dedication to, zero preventable harm continues to help save patient lives around the world. He was the co-inventor of what is now recognized as "modern pulse oximetry," a non-invasive technology that reduces patient harm in hospitals and homes.

Arriving at Angel Stadium in Anaheim, I led the team in a moment of appreciation for Alicia Cole, a PSMF board member, victim of repeated medical errors and associated morbidities, and a staunch fighter for the elimination of preventable harm. Alicia had been a successful actress, often playing the role of a physician on TV.

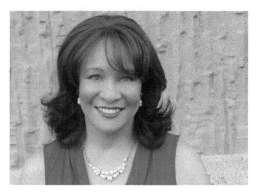

Alicia Cole
Photo courtesy of Alicia Cole

Alicia was gracious in sending me her story:

"There's no need for a second opinion. I'm the best infectious disease specialist in the valley, probably the state. No one else is going to tell you anything different," and

with that the doctor walked out of the room leaving me and my visiting friends, Tammy and Barbie, to stare at one another in disbelief.

For the next two days, the nurses administered my care. As compassionate and attentive as they were, it could not stop the untreated sinus infection and early signs of sepsis from progressing. In his indignation at my asking questions, my doctor refused to order basic lab work and cultures. There were two instances when the nurses gathered my sputum and sinus drainage into a paper cup and tried to submit it to the lab, only to have their efforts rejected because there was no physician order. By the time my patient advocate friends intervened and got the CEO of the hospital to come to my room, it was too late. I was running a fever and starting to have chills. I gently placed the CEO's hand on the hot puffy area on my left hip and explained that the infection had spread through my blood to the weakest part of my body, the site of my prior hospital-acquired infection. I knew what he was feeling was a brewing abscess in my scar tissue.

If my doctor had taken the time to read my medical history, he would have known I had spent the last ten years struggling to recover from multiple hospital-acquired superbugs and flesh-eating disease following a routine procedure. I'd survived near-amputation of my left leg, seven surgeries, nine blood transfusions, three and a half years of care for an open abdominal wound, and ten years of weekly doctor appointments and medical aftercare. I was on the one-yard line of my long drive to recovery when he fumbled the ball. He later admitted he ignored that part of the chart since I only had a "simple sinus infection." He never apologized.

I'm one of the lucky ones. I survived this experience after two more surgeries, two more blood transfusions, blood clots in both arms from central-line infections, another two years with an open healing hip wound, depression, and PTSD (post-traumatic stress disorder).

A culture of patient safety starts with a foundation of ethical responsibility and respect for patients and coworkers to protect patients from preventable harm.

Later that day, we headed back to Chapman University and completed our ten-mile loop. During dinner that evening, Cathy and I debated on whether we should drive to San Francisco and Oakland. The third COVID spike was now out of control, daily infection rates almost double from what they were the previous week. The presidential election was three days away, both of us nervous about protests and riots in large cities, depending on the outcome. We had already been caught in the middle of too many uprisings in cities we walked through this past summer, so we decided to skip northern California and drive back to Phoenix, preferring to be safe at home on election night.

After nine straight months, I walked almost 1,700 miles, visiting twenty Major League ballparks, twelve spring training facilities, and three minor league stadiums. I realized I wasn't going to visit the ten remaining Major League cities before I finished in Jacksonville Beach, Florida. The pandemic was getting worse and experts predicted an exponential growth of infection rates during the upcoming holiday season. The "show" would have to wait until 2021.

"To forget the dead would be akin to killing them a second time."

Elie Weisel

Monday, November 8th, 2020

Miles walked = 1,769
Steps = 4,142,456

I began to feel emotionally drained and wanted to isolate myself from the craziness I witnessed during my walk—1,769 miles bearing witness to political polarity, division, and racial unrest. Now, less than a week after the votes were counted, claims of voter fraud and a stolen election continued to dominate the headlines.

Adding to the political and social media insanity, pandemic infection rates were skyrocketing. On November 1st, the number of new U.S. COVID cases per day hit 74,000, two and a half times greater than the highest number of new infection cases during the first spike in April and higher than any day during the second surge last July. While others were willing to board airplanes, hop on trains, or drive to visit friends and family for the holidays, I opted to stay locked down in Phoenix.

Walking has always had a calming effect on me. Similar to the loneliness of the long-distance runner, my rhythm of walking has a way of generating a harmonic for my thinking and reflective time. As my steps increase, my thoughts follow suit and I begin to notice everything of beauty and wonder around me: hummingbirds with their brilliant flashes of colors and their amazing energy. Jackrabbits scampering across the rocky desert floor, suddenly leaping six feet into the air like a bouncing furry ball, fleeing my approaching footsteps. The saguaro cacti that flank my path with their three-inch spines protecting them against animals, hot and cold temperatures, and breaking up the air flow to reduce evaporation. The century-old cacti can have nine to ten branches coming off the central trunk with baseball-size holes in their sides, the beak of desert birds pecking through the cactus' hard shell, creating a nesting place for their young. This is my therapy, the thought of finishing this challenge seemed not only achievable, but inevitable.

By Thanksgiving weekend, the number of miles walked jumped to 1,900, virtually passing through Mississippi and into southern Alabama on my way to the Atlantic Ocean. But as my total walking mileage increased, so did the number of new COVID cases, hitting 177,858 U.S. citizens per day. The number of hospitalizations, ICU admissions, and deaths across the country also continued to increase, COVID deaths now over 1,400 patients per day. Hospitals and healthcare workers were bracing for the carnage heading their way.

On December 18th, daily COVID infections broke 250,000, more than a million new cases per week with 3,000 deaths per day, the highest daily mortality rate since the pandemic began nine months ago. By mid-December, I had walked over 2,000 miles, which put me forty miles from the Florida panhandle. Was my daily obsession of placing one foot in front of another competing on some level with the high numbers of COVID-19 cases? Were each of my steps dedicated to those who died of COVID, to those who lost loved ones, to patients who were long haulers with severe side effects, and to the dedicated healthcare workers who gave their lives to care for patients?

With a possible end in sight, I began thinking about the remainder of my walk across America as four one-hundred-mile segments. Maintaining my daily walking mileage, I had five ten-day segments left, the lower numbers sounding even easier. I calculated an arrival in Jacksonville sometime between February 18th and 20th, 2021.

In early January, I got in line, rolled up my sleeve, and received my first dose of the COVID vaccine, scheduling my second dose four weeks later. I was now fully vaccinated. The early vaccine data looked strong, showing those who received both doses of the vaccine had a lower chance of contracting the virus. If they did get infected, vaccinated people had milder symptoms and few were getting seriously ill or dying. At this point, I felt more comfortable flying to Jacksonville, and finishing my walk on the white sands of the Atlantic.

The third COVID spike plateaued in early February. People began lining up in droves to receive their first vaccination at outpatient facilities or make-shift clinics, mainly large stadium parking lots. I now felt safe enough to book a flight to complete my last walks in Jacksonville, Florida.

Breaking in my twelfth pair of running shoes, the realization hit me: my challenge ends soon. I kept thinking about the end game, the climax, of my walk across America, and the huge local, regional, and national impact it has had for the patient safety movement—for all patients and caregivers who have suffered preventable harm.

I kept saying, "Run, Forrest, Run." Thinking back to that early *Forrest Gump* movie when my wine-driven idea of walking across the country first originated, I would have given myself less than a one in one thousand chance of completing the walk because of my age and personal health issues, not to mention the pandemic and surrounding racial injustice erupting across the country. It was baseball that kept my spirits high but it was raising awareness about healthcare safety that drove me to finish. Babe Ruth, "The Bambino," once said, "Never let the fear of striking out keep you from playing the game."

When I arrived in Jacksonville Florida on February 16th, the weather was perfect; temperatures stayed in the low seventies with a cool breeze off the ocean—the perfect environment for walking. There were thirty-one miles left before reaching my goal of 2,452 miles, which meant I needed to average ten miles per day over three days.

I started walking early Monday, stopping first for my usual jolt of caffeine, a cup of Starbucks' clover-brewed Sumatra roast. After belting down half a cup, my legs seemed to move at a faster pace, like gliding through the air, and for the first time since late summer my body didn't hurt. No aches or pains in my hips or knees. No stiffness in my back. I was wired.

Jacksonville, or Jax, no longer smells like a pulp mill. It's hip, young, fit, and green. The young people who grew up under the stigma of the stench and sprawl returned to transform Jax into a unique city with a thriving art, music, and historic neighborhoods, including the childhood home of Lynyrd Skynyrd. And don't forget the NFL's choice to hold the 2005 Super Bowl right here in J-ville.

While walking, I counted the number of people wearing masks on one hand despite the reality of 500,000-plus U.S. COVID deaths. I passed hash houses with crowds lined up waiting to be seated. Strip malls dot both sides of Ocean Boulevard with tattoo parlors and souvenir stores selling postcards, T-shirts, beach towels, gooey suntan lotions, and plastic sunglasses, along with pails, shovels, and beach balls.

My pedometer shows a total of twelve miles. I don't want to stop. An hour later, I surpass fifteen miles and still feel energetic. I kept going. Sixty minutes later, my Fitbit displays 18.5 miles and says in black letters, "Enough for today." Three hundred and fifty-three straight days of walking, and I established a new personal best.

My goal for Tuesday was to walk eight or nine miles. Heading south on Ponte Vedra Boulevard, the sidewalk was my own. I walked past Spanish- and Mediterranean-style beachfront estates with white stone and marble exteriors, two-story sculptured columns, twelve-foot mahogany doors, and rows of palm trees lining gated driveways. An occasional ultramodern home built of steel with two-story glass panels seemed disruptive and out of place. The opposite side of the boulevard was lined with high-end country clubs, each with sculptured fairways, manicured greens, and strategically placed small lakes, making me wonder how many lakes were homes to alligators.

After dinner, I spent the rest of the evening getting ready for the final day. I had arranged for 200 orange "Unite for Safe Care" flags to be shipped to Jacksonville Beach so I could plant them on the beach my last day, along with a two-foot by three-foot poster displaying faces of children, spouses, parents, grandparents—all lost to preventable medical harm. Using a black ink Sharpie, I sat on the bed and began printing each of their names on the flags.

Michael Skolnik, Lewis Blackman, Yogiraj Bates, Alyssa Hemmelgarn, Grant Lars Visscher, Drew Hughes, Judie Burrows, Pat Sheridan, Louise Batz.

Children, spouses, and parents who died needlessly from preventable medical harm.

Josh Nahum, Gabby Galbo, Lola Fitch, Noah Lord, Alicia Cole, Nile Moss, Pat Denton, Lily Blackburn, Jack Gentry.

An empty chair at the dinner table on Thanksgiving and Christmas.

Josie King, Michelle Ballog, Karen Coughlin, Rory Staunton, Jennifer Neiberger, Rory Freeman, Joshua Titcombe, Abdi Towfigh.

Each day of my walk, I remembered one of these beautiful people who died because of preventable medical harm.

Adrienne Cullen, Chris Salazar, Nora Bostrom, Noah McGrath, Michael Seres, Bill Aydt, Emily Jerry.

I thought about how long it would take to write 250,000-plus names on individual flags.

Parker Stewart, Toby Hudson, Collin Haller, Don Newton, Sam Moorish, Glenn Saarinen, Josh Barron.

I finished writing 200 total tonight, each name on the back of a flag. And it took me over an hour.

Over the course of my one-year walk across the country, another 250,000 patients lost their lives because of preventable medical harm. The reality of losing a quarter of a million people in the span of 365 days and the fact that there are many more unreported errors is overwhelming, inexcusable, and unacceptable.

Lying in bed, the names written on the flags kept running through my thoughts like numbers on a New York Stock Exchange tote board, each name followed by another and then another. Their loss and the never-ending pain inflicted needlessly on families had me tossing and turning for three hours before finally falling asleep.

I woke up Wednesday morning to a chilly hotel room from a cold front that passed through during the night dropping morning temperatures into the low fifties. The normally sunny skies had been replaced with ominous grey clouds, making me believe rain was imminent. To make the day worse, a twenty-five- to thirty-mile an hour wind was coming off the water, causing the wind chill temperature to feel twenty degrees colder. I dressed in a light sweatshirt, long running pants, and my Javy Baez Cubs jersey.

I felt the chill of the wind, like a slap across the face, as I stepped through the hotel's sliding glass doors. It was brutal, the coldest day I had experienced walking over the last year—my breath visible every time I exhaled. For the first time, my face mask provided more than just protection from the virus.

Unlike the previous two days of walking, the streets and strip malls were empty as the tourists from the north opted to stay inside their hotel rooms. Walking east on Beach Boulevard, Michael, a photographer hired by the PSMF, spotted me crossing the bridge connecting Jacksonville with Jacksonville Beach.

"Are you Dr. Mayer?" he shouted while standing at the back of his car. His gray Jacksonville Jaguar sweatshirt and hooded leather coat made me wish I was the photographer today and he was the walker.

"I am, and please call me Dave," I shouted back from about ten feet away, my voice competing with the gusting winds. "Is this really Florida or am I back in Chicago?" I added.

I walked the last mile down Beach Boulevard with a combination of sadness and elation. The low came from saying goodbye to my year of walking across America. And the high from completing this improbable challenge.

Michael was capturing every step as he clicked away, taking more than a hundred pictures over a five-minute span, like I was a fashion model walking down a runway. As I crossed Third Street, I could see the boardwalk entrance to the beachfront. Walking past the Four Points Sheraton Hotel and down the boardwalk, I could not believe it was over. Three hundred and fifty-five straight days of walking over 2,452 miles and 5,527,991 steps.

I shed my running shoes and socks about twenty feet from the water. I rolled my pant legs up above my knees and walked the remaining steps to the ocean. As I reached the edge of the water, something took me back to that February evening over a year ago watching the movie *Forrest Gump*. I thought about the scene when Forrest turned to the crowd of people running behind him, and I turned to Michael and said, "I'm pretty tired...I think I will go home."

As I entered the water, the waves of an icy-cold Atlantic Ocean splashed against my bare legs, but I didn't care. Nothing would ruin this last day.

After walking back to shore, I headed to the hotel parking lot and retrieved the one-hundred-picture poster, and the 200 orange flags from the trunk of my rental car. Finding an area protected from the thirty-mile-an-hour wind gusts, Michael helped me place all 200 flags on the beach and secure the poster.

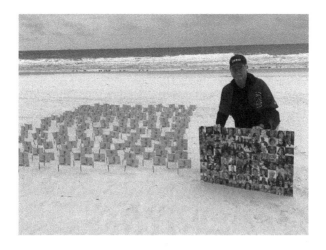

My last memorial ceremony on the beach was not for one child, one parent, one grandparent, or one spouse as I had done the previous 354 days. It was for everyone, patients and caregivers, who lost their lives this past year, for those we lost in previous years, and unfortunately for those still to come. With the wind gusting around us, Michael and I lowered our heads in a moment of silence before exchanging hugs and saying goodbye.

I headed south for my five-hour drive to Fort Lauderdale where I would meet up with my family. Thirty minutes into the drive, something peculiar occurred. My body and mind felt like someone had pulled the plug, what little energy and emotion I had left slowly exiting my body like beads of perspiration. Exiting the highway, I pulled into a Starbucks parking lot, turned the car off, and closed my eyes. It finally hit me—the 3:30am wake-ups, the Arizona desert heat, the thick Midwest humidity, the fingers pointed in my face, the broken glass littering the sidewalks, the aches and pains in my knees, hips and back, and the names of those lost. Like a marathon runner at mile twenty, I hit the wall. After a forty-five-minute nap and a much-needed caffeine load, I continued driving south, deciding to make two more stops along the way.

One was at Clover Park, the spring training ballpark of the New York Mets and the second at Roger Dean Stadium in Jupiter, Florida, the spring training facility of the Miami Marlins and St. Louis Cardinals. How could a baseball junkie miss an opportunity to visit two more baseball parks?

Staring at the empty seats at both stadiums brought back memories of Wrigley Field on the Near North Side in Chicago, where I grew up. I close my eyes and I'm there listening to Pat Pieper. His career began in 1916 when the Cubs moved to Weeghman Park, which later became Wrigley Field. At that time, Pieper would run up and down the aisles with a fourteen-pound megaphone sharing the starting line-ups for both teams. An electronic public address system was installed in 1932, allowing Pieper to sit in a booth and share the starting line-ups before the game. I used to imagine him announcing my name, Attention!...Attention!...David Mayer! Have your pencil...and scorecard ready...and I'll give you the lineup...I even recall when in 1961 he got to throw out the first ball to open the season, after which he reported to work as usual, in his chair behind home plate, making his announcements, and providing fresh baseballs to the plate umpire.

Wrigleyville was my playground whenever I scored tickets to a ballgame and there were plenty of those days. It wasn't just the game I enjoyed, but also the lovely frame where it all took place, which can't be said about all stadiums.

I'm thinking about all those empty seats at Wrigley Field, all 40,000, 16 percent, or about one-sixth of the people who die each year from preventable medical harm. I'm not done yet. I'm only in the seventh inning stretch and there's a lot of baseball left to play. My next challenge focuses on filling up those 40,000 seats and celebrating one day every season, maybe September 17th, calling it Patient and Healthcare Worker Safety Day. I imagine looking up and hearing the roar of the crowd and seeing bright-colored orange banners waving in the wind, high pitched cheers coming from the grandstands, bleachers, box seats, suites, upper and lower decks, dugouts, and even the players on the field, whooping it up for Patient and Healthcare Worker Safety Day!

I'll still be walking daily, focusing my thoughts and energy on this new challenge and continuing to raise awareness for patients and caregivers who die each year from preventable medical errors, and for healthcare professionals who face escalating workplace injuries, depression, burnout, and suicide rates. And at the finale, I'll be part of the crowd at Wrigley, walking along with all the other healthcare safety advocates, holding up our banners, marching around the bases to the tune of "Take me out to the Ballgame."

Let this book be a renewed call to action so we can better protect those who provide care, as well as those who receive care within our health system.

If my walking saves one life, it's worth every step.

Epilogue: "The Club"

> "To the family we are born with and the family
> we make along the way."
>
> *Leslie Higgins; Ted Lasso TV show*

I walked 2,460 miles over 355 consecutive days in memory of hundreds lost to preventable medical harm.

There are two people I never acknowledged. They walked with me every step of the way, but their names were never painted on a rock with bright colors or mentioned at memorial services or during moments of silence. And even though their spirits remain tattooed in my heart, I never shared their stories, their distinct personalities, or their struggles. The errors involved concerning their standard of care were never talked about—not until now. In fact, I rarely discussed that part of my life with anyone.

It's always been difficult to focus on those memories because of a fear of revealing my own shortcomings—a guilt for not acting as their medical advocate and for not saving them from unnecessary pain and suffering.

This book is not complete without including who they were and what happened to them. Their names are Ben Mayer and Debbie Mayer—my father and sister, both victims of a compromised healthcare system.

In October of 1996, at the age of seventy-four, my father was diagnosed with Non-Hodgkin lymphoma. Unlike my mother, he had always been in excellent health—no heart disease, no diabetes, "all systems go," as he used to say. His good health amazed me because he never exercised, ate whatever junk food he wanted, and remained thin as a pole. Despite the cancer diagnosis, he was upbeat and confident he could beat it.

The pathologist report showed a rare form of lymphoma, referred to as mantle cell lymphoma. With my father's good health, the oncologist thought he had a 90 percent cure rate. I first became skeptical about the diagnosis after consulting with physicians in Chicago. His blood tests were consistent with a more common diffuse large B-cell lymphoma, but when I shared my concerns with his oncologist, he assured me the original diagnosis was correct.

After placement of a central venous port, my father began receiving chemo cocktails three days a week, for six weeks, specifically for treating his mantle lymphoma. I flew to Fort Lauderdale the second week of his treatments to check on his progress and keep him company, wanting to be there for him just as he was always there for my mother. Unlike my mother's cancer journey fourteen years prior, when I was a fourth-year medical student, I was now a senior-level physician and felt more confident speaking with the physicians and nurses leading his care.

I drove him to the health center, following his directions to a part of town that didn't look familiar. When I reached a strip mall, my father pointed toward a one-story windowless storefront situated between a tattoo parlor and a 7-Eleven. Parking his car, I asked, "Is this where you receive your treatments?" I had expected a modern ambulatory care facility located adjacent to a hospital—not a rundown building looking like it needed demolition.

With a weak nod, he turned to me and said, "This is where I go for chemo. I just follow the doctor's orders."

The center had no windows. It was colorless, with dingy walls void of pictures, making me feel as if I had entered a morgue in the basement of a hospital. After checking in, the nurse led my father to a stained blue tweed recliner alongside ten other cancer patients sitting in a semi-circle, three feet apart with no curtains or dividing walls between them. I watched as nurses struggled, trying to squeeze between patients to start or change IV infusion bags. It was apparent from the number of treatment chairs, the condition of the building, and room setup, that financial gain trumped safety, patient experience, and outcomes.

During the third week of treatment, my father's port site became red and painful, serous fluid oozing through the dressing, the infection necessitating removal and replacement of his port, along with a course of antibiotics. Three weeks later, my father spiked a fever of 102 degrees. It wasn't long before his new port became infected. Blood cultures soon confirmed the infection had now entered his bloodstream. The second port was removed and replaced, along with another round of antibiotics, but he continued to suffer from high fevers and periods of chills. His shaky hands had trouble holding onto a glass of water without spilling. After a battery of tests, searching for the source of his infection, a cardiac echo revealed bacterial endocarditis which required six weeks of IV antibiotics. My father's two central line catheter infections were devastating to me. As a cardiac anesthesiologist, I placed central line catheters every day and knew how easy infections occur if best practices are not followed. Waking up in the middle of the night, I started punishing myself for failing my father and not taking a more active role in his care, believing I could have prevented his bacterial endocarditis.

Whenever I talked with him on the phone, his voice couldn't hide the depression and frustration he was feeling. There were moments of silence and a few times I thought I heard him crying. He kept asking, "What more could go wrong?"

His lymphoma wasn't responding to chemotherapy. Instead, it continued to spread throughout his body. His oncologist began questioning whether the pathologist's assessment was correct. I wished I had trusted my gut, listened to colleagues, pushed my concerns, and asked for a second or third opinion before my father started his treatments.

Flying into Fort Lauderdale Airport over the years became routine; I knew the flight routes, the cities we passed; Louisville, Knoxville, Athens, Valdosta. I learned the time it took from take-off to landing (two hours and thirty-two minutes in the air), a distance of 1,169 miles, 1,882 kilometers, or 1,016 nautical miles. Depending on the winds, sometimes we circled in off the ocean and other times we vectored over the Everglades.

My stepmother, Lilly, greeted me at the door of their apartment and led me to the bedroom, where I found a thin man, a shadow of himself, wasting away. He was lying in bed, looking pale, with pillows propped up all around him, as if he might hurt himself if he rolled to one side. It reminded me of my mother's last days. He had lost twenty pounds since I saw him a month ago. His dark black lines under his eyes and sunken cheek bones resembled a skeleton that hung in my anatomy lab.

Father tried to smile, somehow finding the strength to reach out and clasp my hand in his. He looked defeated and scared. The spirit and fight I was used to seeing were gone. The last time I saw my mother before she died, I needed to stay strong for my father, refusing to cry in front of him. This time I leaned down, still holding on to his hand, and we wept together.

A few weeks later, the hospice nurse called letting Cathy know my father didn't have long to live. Hospice nurses have an acute sense of knowing when patients are close to death. I was on a flight back to Chicago from San Francisco where I had given a patient safety talk. Walking off the plane, my cell phone lit up. It was Cathy, letting me know my father was dying. She booked me on a flight from Chicago to Miami leaving in an hour.

Lilly and I hugged as I entered their apartment. I walked into the living room where my father's hospital bed was set up, allowing my stepmother a quiet bedroom for sleep. Dad looked peaceful lying in bed under a dark brown blanket that covered his body from the neck down. His respirations were shallow and rapid. A nasal cannula wrapped around his face, providing oxygen to his failing body. I bent down to kiss him on the forehead. He stayed motionless and was unresponsive to my voice. I glanced at the pulse oximeter monitor on a table in the corner of a dimly lit living room, the only light coming from a lamp next to the sofa. The annoying monitor beeped with each heartbeat, and his blood oxygen saturation of "94" flashed on the screen. I removed the hissing cannula from his face telling the nurse, "There's no need for this anymore." I wanted to end his agony and make his last few hours more comfortable.

Reaching into a cabinet drawer, I pulled out a disc and placed it in the player next to his bed. It was a Mandy Patinkin CD I had bought for him a few months before. My father loved listening to Patinkin singing famous songs in Yiddish, my favorite being, "Take Me Out to the Ballgame." It served as a distraction to his persistent pain. Dad and I listened to it that night until he died in the early hours of the morning, with me at his bedside, holding his hand with my finger tip on his radial artery. I watched his agonal breathing—the classic sign of death. Looking at the hospice nurse, holding back tears and not sure why, I shared what she already knew—I was the doctor who pronounced my father dead.

At his funeral, I placed the Patinkin CD in his coffin before shutting it one last time.

My sister, Debbie, died in 2008, at forty-nine years of age. She was driving when a car ran a stop sign, hitting the passenger side. A trip to the emergency room revealed two broken ribs on her lower right side but no other injuries. While the broken ribs were painful, Debbie never complained. She was discharged from the emergency department with no further follow-up.

For the next ten days, my sister complained of increased discomfort—an extreme pain located in the upper right quadrant, different from her original injury. When she followed up with her doctor, she was told broken ribs take weeks to heal and there was no need for further testing or evaluation. I suggested she request a scan of the area, knowing that lower rib fractures can cause trauma to the kidneys, liver, or spleen, but Debbie didn't want to push her doctor and said nothing. Two days later, she spiked a fever of 104 degrees and had uncontrolled vomiting before she lost consciousness and was rushed to the hospital. Debbie was admitted to the ICU in septic shock. A scan revealed a large hematoma (collection of blood), most likely a result of a liver laceration, hidden above the liver and below the right diaphragm. Her infection spread quicker than anyone expected, shutting down her kidney and liver function within hours. Debbie was too sick to be taken to the operating room, so we all prayed the antibiotics and supportive care would treat the infection.

The next morning, Cathy and I flew to Fort Lauderdale. We met Ron, Debbie's husband, in the ICU. By then, Debbie's kidney and liver had failed, and her lungs were full of fluid filling her endotracheal tube with pink frothy fluid, requiring constant suctioning. She was in DIC (disseminated intra-vascular coagulation), an end-of-life systemic clotting disorder that disrupts blood flow. Her intravenous lines began to bleed at each puncture site. I sat at her bedside that evening, watching the monitor show beats of ventricular ectopy, which led to a slowing of her heart rate, then long pauses of no beats before flatlining. For days, I kept beating myself up for not pushing Debbie to get an abdominal scan.

For years, I struggled knowing that the last two members of my imme-diate family had died—my father and my only sister, both from preventable harm, leaving me the lone survivor. To this day, I still punish myself for not being more present and vocal at that time in my life.

I have kept the stories about the deaths of my father and sister to myself. Others share their personal losses to heal, improve patient safety, and to leave a legacy for their loved one. They are more courageous than I am and deserve the podium. Those are the true heroes of patient safety.

Families who have lost loved ones to preventable medical harm say the pain never goes away. My grandparents and parents taught me well—leave the past in the past and live in the present. I have chosen to keep the pain inside and move on, knowing the pain will always be there, using my role as a phy-sician and healthcare leader to create change and make care safer.